Unlocking Nature's Secrets: The Power of Oils

Ancient Remedies for Modern Living

Olivia Bennett

Table of Contents

INTRODUCTION

In today's society, which is characterized by the prevalence of contemporary medicine and technology in our health and wellness routines, traditional remedies are enjoying a significant return in popularity. This is a positive development. Essential oils have become increasingly popular in recent years due to their natural potential to cure, calm, and rejuvenate. This is in addition to the time-honored traditions that have been practiced for centuries. This surge in popularity, on the other hand, is not merely a transitory fad; rather, it is a reawakening of the power that nature has kept throughout the course of history. The book "Unlocking Nature's Secrets: The Power of Oils: Ancient Remedies for Modern Living" takes readers on a journey through time, analyzing the historical significance of essential oils as well as their place in our modern lives. The book will take readers on a journey through time.

The use of essential oils dates back to ancient civilizations such as Egypt, Greece, and China, where they were initially utilized. Essential oils have been utilized for a long amount of time, with their roots extending back to ancient times. These civilizations made use of oils not just for therapeutic purposes but also for the purpose of performing religious rites, assisting spiritual healing, and providing regular cosmetic care. Oils were also used for the goal of providing regular cosmetic care. Since ancient times, these potent plant extracts have been revered for their restorative properties and transformative potential. This can be seen in everything from Cleopatra's beauty rituals to the ancient Greeks' use of oils for therapeutic massages. On the other hand, as time progressed and the development of new pharmaceuticals progressed, the utilization of natural oils in conventional medical practices became less popular. At this time, people are looking for natural alternatives that are in harmony with the body and are going back to these traditional therapies.

Discovering the cultural, spiritual, and therapeutic functions that essential oils have played over the course of the ages is the subject of this book, which dives into the historical context of essential oils. It shows the ways in which classic extraction procedures, like as steam distillation and cold pressing, were developed and perfected in order to produce oils that harness the full strength of the plants from which they are produced. When we have a better understanding of the history of essential oils, we are better able to appreciate their significance not only in traditional medicine but also in the natural health movement that is taking place now.

Essential oils, on the other hand, are not merely remnants of the past. Aromatherapy, cosmetics, and even integrative medical procedures have helped them rediscover their role in the present era for which they were originally developed. This book examines the scientific rationale underlying the efficacy of essential oils, with a particular emphasis on the chemical composition of these oils and the ways in which they interact with the body. Recent scientific research has demonstrated that the molecules included in essential oils have the ability to influence the neural system, in addition to alleviating pain, reducing inflammation, and even improving mental well-being. By bridging the gap between old knowledge and modern study, these discoveries have provided a thorough understanding of the functioning of essential oils.

In addition to the scientific principles, "Unlocking Nature's Secrets" provides actionable advice on how to include essential oils into your everyday routine. Essential oils have a wide range of uses that can improve both physical and mental well-being. These applications include both the alleviation of stress and anxiety as well as the enhancement of your beauty routine. If you want to treat common conditions, strengthen your immune system, or simply create an environment that is peaceful, this book provides easy-to-follow suggestions on how to utilize essential oils in a way that is both safe and effective.

The central purpose of "Unlocking Nature's Secrets" is to equip you with the tools necessary to reestablish a connection with the natural world. When we live in a culture that is driven by synthetics and fast-paced, essential oils, serve as a reminder that nature has potent remedies to many of the difficulties that we face in the present day. It is possible for us to regain a sense of equilibrium, healing, and vigor in our lives by rediscovering these old medicines and utilizing the ageless wisdom that they contain. In this book, you will learn how to unleash the power of oils, which are traditional treatments that can help you live a healthy life in our modern age.

CHAPTER I

The Historical Use of Essential Oils

Ancient Civilizations

Investigating the usage of essential oils in ancient societies is one way to uncover the fundamental link that exists between nature and human well-being that is unchanged by the passage of time. This relationship is unaffected by the passage of time. Essential oils, which are concentrated extracts from plants, have been revered for their therapeutic properties, spiritual significance, and practical applications for thousands of years. Essential oils are derived from plants. In many different ancient communities, these oils were not only believed to be instruments for the purpose of medical healing, but they were also considered to be sacred substances that had the capacity to improve spiritual practices, beauty rituals, and even social standing. This was the case in many of the societies that existed in the past. It is possible to trace the origins of essential oils back to ancient civilizations such as Egypt, Mesopotamia, Greece, Rome, India, and China. This reveals a thorough awareness of natural therapies and the function that they play in the day-to-day lives of people. There is a common thread that binds all communities together, and that is the underlying veneration for the power of plants to heal and transform. It is not the oils themselves that serve as the unifying factor that binds different cultures together, despite the fact that every civilization has developed its own distinctive method of making use of these oils.

Essential oils were utilized in a substantial manner throughout the entirety of ancient Egypt, not only in everyday life but also in sacred events. There is a possibility that the Egyptians were the first culture to develop sophisticated methods for extracting oils from plants. Within the context of this society, the utilization of essential oils embraced a wide variety of applications, reaching far beyond the area of purely therapeutic use. Essential components of their religious ceremonies and burial rites included the use of oils such as frankincense, myrrh, cedarwood, and lotus. The use of these oils was also performed. Those who held this belief believed that the fragrant qualities of oils had the capacity to establish a connection between the living and the divine, so bridging the gap between the physical and spiritual realms. One type of frankincense, in particular, was utilized for the purpose of embalming the deceased as well as being burned as incense during religious rites. There was a widespread notion that the application of oils of this kind assisted in preparing the soul for its passage into the hereafter. Further evidence of the spiritual significance that the Egyptians put on oils is shown by the extensive use of oils in the process of mummification, which involved the embalming of bodies and wrapping them in linens that had been soaked in aromatic substances. Additionally, essential oils were utilized in the cosmetic and beauty rituals of the day, in addition to their spiritual significance. It was stated that Cleopatra, one of the most famous individuals in Egyptian history, had a special fondness for jasmine and rose oil, both of which she utilized to enhance her appearance and attractiveness. Additionally, oils were utilized for personal grooming purposes, such as in perfumes, bath routines, and even as bug repellents, which exemplifies the wide range of applications that oils have in everyday life.

The use of essential oils has been documented beginning as far back as 3,000 BCE in Mesopotamia, which is considered to be the cradle of civilization. The ancient Sumerians preserved clay tablets that contained allusions to oils such as cypress and myrrh. These oils were utilized in the treatment of medical conditions and for the purpose of anointing the body. Following in the footsteps of the Sumerians, the Babylonians brought about an expansion of the use of essential oils in religious rites. They believed that the fragrant characteristics of these oils could cleanse both the body and the soul. During the process of entering temples, it was common practice to use oils to cleanse and prepare worshippers. This was done to ensure that they were spiritually pure before encountering their gods. Essential oils were utilized in religious and medical rituals by the Assyrians, another civilization that existed in the region at the same time. The fact that their medicinal books were written on clay tablets demonstrates that they had a profound understanding of aromatherapy and herbalism. Historically, it was normal practice to employ oils derived from cedarwood and juniper for the purpose of treating respiratory ailments, skin conditions, and even psychological illnesses such as anxiety and depression. This early realization of the mind-body connection, in which aromatic oils were employed to relieve both physical maladies and mental disturbance, exemplifies a holistic approach to healing that would lead to the influence of other cultures in the future.

Building on the knowledge that had been passed down from the Egyptians and Mesopotamians, the ancient Greeks took a scientific approach to the usage of essential oils as they moved westward. Hippocrates, who is considered to be the "father" of modern medicine, was a staunch supporter of the usage of essential oils for therapeutic purposes, notably in the context of massages and hydrotherapy. He was of the opinion that aromatic oils had the potential to improve health by cleansing both the body and the mind. Essential oils were also utilized in the medical practices of Greek physicians such as Galen, who wrote extensively about the effects that essential oils had on the body because of their use. Lavandin, rosemary, and thyme were among the oils that were frequently utilized due to the antibacterial and therapeutic capabilities that they possessed. Athletes from Greece, particularly those who were competing in the Olympic Games, massaged their muscles with oils in the mistaken belief that doing so would improve their strength and endurance. Essential oils were highly esteemed not only for their medical applications but also for the meaningful part they played in the religious practices of the Greeks. Since it was believed that the perfume of burning incense carried petitions to the gods, temples were frequently filled with the aroma of burning incense. Essential oils were used by the Greeks, much like they were by the Egyptians, to improve their spiritual experiences. The Greeks believed that there was a connection between the aromatic world of plants and the divine presence.

It is possible to observe the influence of Greek methods in ancient Rome, where essential oils were utilized for both health and luxury purposes. The lavish use of oils and scents in Roman baths, which were an essential part of Roman society, earned them a legendary reputation. When it came to maintaining one's bodily and mental well-being, the Romans felt that cleanliness and health were inextricably linked, and they considered bathing to be an indispensable component of this process. Immediately following a bath, Romans would rub themselves with olive oil that had been infused with fragrant herbs like rosemary and lavender. This was done not just for the therapeutic advantages of the herbs but also for their aroma. Additionally, it was common practice for Roman troops to bring essential oils into combat with them, where they were utilized to cure wounds and increase morale. In addition to relaxing the thoughts of warriors before and after the battle, oils such as myrrh and frankincense were utilized to disinfect wounds, hasten the healing process, and speed up the healing process. Essential oils were used to treat a wide variety of ailments and conditions, and Roman physicians proceeded to expand their use of essential oils by building on the knowledge of medicine that they had gained from the Greeks. In the same way that the Greeks did, the Romans recognized the spiritual significance of oils and made use of them in their temples and during religious rituals in order to show respect for their deities.

The usage of aromatic plants and the extracts of those plants was thriving in the East, particularly in India and China, at the same time that Western civilizations were expanding their knowledge of essential oils. The ancient Indian medical method known as Ayurveda, which has been in use for more than five thousand years, included the use of essential oils as an essential component. Sandalwood, turmeric, and jasmine are some of the oils that Ayurvedic practitioners utilize to improve physical, emotional, and spiritual health by balancing the doshas, or forces, of the body. For the purpose of treating a wide variety of diseases, including digestive disorders and skin issues, these oils were utilized in the form of massages, inhalations, and as components of herbal remedies. Sandalwood, in particular, was considered to have profound spiritual importance. Because of its calming and grounding characteristics, it was frequently utilized in religious rites and meditation techniques. In India, essential oils were also utilized in the treatment of beauty issues, notably by women who would apply aromatic oils to their skin in order to improve their appearance and attract positive energy. Essential oils were not only a type of physical medicine but also a tool for reaching spiritual enlightenment, according to the Indian understanding of essential oils, which was profoundly connected with their philosophical and spiritual beliefs.

In ancient China, essential oils were closely associated with traditional Chinese medicine (TCM), which is a healthcare system that aims to achieve a balance between the yin and yang energies that are present in the body. Traditional Chinese herbalists devised complex methods for extracting oils from plants and employing these oils in the treatment of a wide range of illnesses. Ginger, cinnamon, and tea tree oil were among the herbs that were frequently utilized for the purpose of enhancing circulation, combating infections, and bolstering the immune system. In addition, the Chinese thought that essential oils had the ability to affect the flow of qi, which is the vital force that flows through the body. They utilized essential oils in conjunction with acupuncture and other therapies in order to bolster health and vitality. In addition, essential oils had a significant role in the spiritual activities of the Chinese people. These oils were utilized in spiritual practices such as meditation and the burning of incense to provide an atmosphere that was conducive to the development of spirituality. The Chinese approach to essential oils was comprehensive, treating both the physical and spiritual requirements of the individual. This method was similar to China's approach to essential oils in India.

There is a profound link between people and the natural environment, as evidenced by the ancient civilizations' veneration of essential oils. These societies understood that plants possessed the ability to cure, transform, and elevate the human experience with their medicinal properties. Essential oils played a crucial part in defining the lives and beliefs of these ancient peoples, being utilized in a variety of contexts, including religious rites, medical treatments, and daily grooming. In the modern essential oil market, where the knowledge of the ancients continues to inform our understanding of plant-based therapy, the methods that they created for extracting and utilizing these oils lay the foundation for the industry.

Considering that we are currently rediscovering these old methods, it is abundantly obvious that the utilization of essential oils is not merely a fleeting fad but rather a continuation of a relationship that has existed between humans and the natural world for a very long time. Essential oils may have been utilized by ancient civilizations for a variety of objectives, yet the fundamental premise behind their use was the same: to harness the force of nature in order to improve one's physical, emotional, and spiritual well-being, respectively. It is a monument to the lasting wisdom of these civilizations and their profound awareness of the healing possibilities of the natural world that essential oils have been passed down from ancient times to the present day.

Traditional Oil Extraction

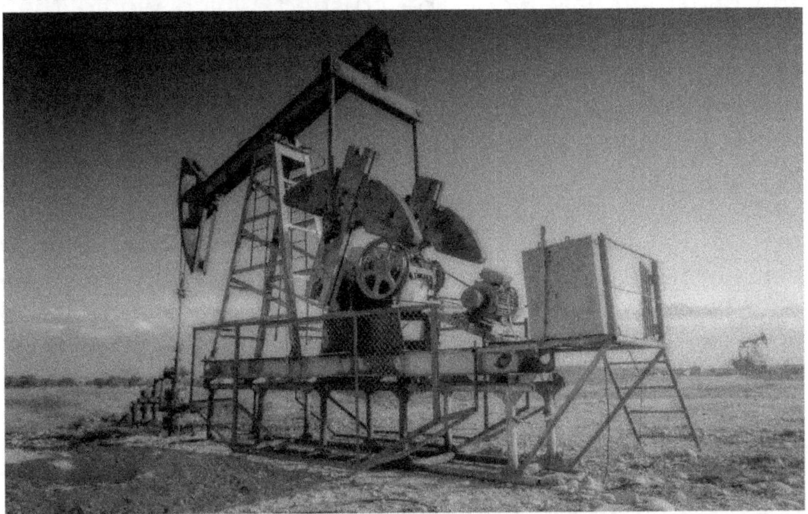

There is a lengthy and complicated history behind the extraction of oil using traditional methods, which are based on old procedures that have been handed down from generation to generation. The process of extracting oil from plants, seeds, nuts, and fruits has seen tremendous improvement throughout the course of history; nonetheless, the fundamental nature of these old processes continues to serve as a tribute to the inventiveness of early civilizations. Traditional oil extraction is not just a method of gaining a lucrative product in many different cultures; it is also a cultural and spiritual exercise that represents respect for nature and the environment. Both of these aspects are important to the culture.

The early techniques for extracting oil were extremely primitive, and they frequently relied on both human ingenuity and the forces of nature. In ancient Egypt, for instance, the process of extracting oil from plants like flaxseed and olives was carried out with the use of straightforward implements such as stone presses and mills that were manually turned. With these early presses, the raw materials would be crushed, which would then result in the release of oil, which would then be collected for usage. The oil that was extracted was frequently utilized in a variety of industries, including the culinary arts, medicine, religious rituals, and the cosmetic industry.

Over the course of several centuries, the method of extracting olive oil has remained practically unaltered in certain places, such as the Mediterranean. Harvesting the olives by hand is followed by crushing them with massive stone wheels or mills as the next step. After the olives have been crushed, the paste that has been generated is put onto mats, which are then layered vertically on top of one another. The oil is forced to flow out of these mats because the weight that is supplied to the mats causes them to be placed in a press. Both the oil's natural flavor and its nutritious benefits are maintained through the use of this approach, which is referred to as the "cold pressing" technique. The use of heat, which can cause the beneficial chemicals in olive oil to degrade, is avoided through the use of cold pressing, which is still the method of choice for generating high-quality olive oil because it is preferred.

Many indigenous civilizations have developed their own distinctive methods of extracting oil from a wide variety of plants, in contrast to the mechanical extraction methods that are used in the Mediterranean region. On the African continent, for instance, the ancient methods of oil extraction frequently entail the processes of boiling and skimming. Extraction of palm oil, which is one of the oils that is used the most in Africa, normally involves boiling the fruit and then removing the oil from the surface of the water after it has been extracted. In addition to being abundant in minerals, the oil that was produced has been a fundamental component of African meals and ceremonies for millennia.

In a similar manner, the extraction of oils from plants such as the coconut and the avocado is typically carried out using physical methods in South American countries. In order to extract the oil from coconuts, for example, the husk is removed, and the flesh is grated before the coconuts are either pressed or boiled. It is well known that the extracted oil, particularly coconut oil, is versatile, as it is utilized in a variety of applications, including cooking, skincare, and traditional medicine. Natural fermentation is another method that is frequently used in certain areas. In this method, the raw materials are allowed to sit and ferment for a period of time, which enables the oil to spontaneously separate from the plant material.

Traditional oil extraction techniques have been used for a very long time in India, which has a long and illustrious Ayurvedic legacy. An extraction technique called "Ghani" pressing is utilized in order to obtain sesame oil, which is an essential component in numerous Ayurvedic medicines. In this method, the sesame seeds are crushed by pressing them through a mill made of stone or wood, which is operated by either animal or human labor. Because of the long grinding process, the oil is able to keep its inherent nutrients and therapeutic capabilities intact without being altered. In a similar manner, the process of extracting coconut oil in southern India often involves drying the coconut flesh (copra) in the sun and then pressing it in order to allow the oil to be extracted. In addition to being profoundly entwined with cultural practices, these traditional approaches are also regarded as a means of establishing a connection with the natural community.

Obtaining essential oils from aromatic plants has also been accomplished through the use of traditional extraction techniques, in addition to the acquisition of edible oils. Techniques for extracting essential oils from flowers, herbs, and spices were established by ancient civilizations such as the Egyptians, Greeks, and Romans. These oils were then utilized in the production of perfumes, medicines, and even in religious ceremonies. The procedure of steam distillation, which is being used today, is one of the oldest methods of extracting essential oils. Steam distillation is a process that involves heating plant materials with steam, which, therefore, causes the volatile oils to evaporate. Following the condensation and collection of the steam and oil vapor, the oil is separated from the water and collected on its own. The delicate perfume of the plant is preserved through the use of this process, which is also frequently utilized in the manufacture of essential oils for aromatherapy and complementary and alternative medicine.

Despite the fact that ancient methods of oil extraction are frequently labor-intensive and time-consuming, they have a number of advantages over modern methods that are designed for industrialization. The inherent properties of the oil are preserved, which is one of the most important advantages obtained. The nutritional value and flavor of the oil may be diminished as a result of the use of contemporary techniques, such as extraction with solvent processing with high temperatures or both. Traditional processes, on the other hand, such as cold pressing and Ghani pressing, are able to maintain the natural vitamins, minerals, and antioxidants that are also present in the oil. This is of utmost significance for oils that are utilized for cosmetic and therapeutic purposes, where the purity and potency of the oil are of utmost importance.

One additional benefit of using conventional methods to extract oil is that they are environmentally friendly. A significant number of these techniques are low-tech and rely on environmentally friendly energy sources, such as human labor or the power of animals. In addition to this, they generate less waste and are less likely to entail the use of dangerous chemicals or additives that are synthetic. In communities where traditional oil extraction is still performed, these practices are frequently regarded as a means of preserving a peaceful relationship with the surrounding environment. In order to ensure the long-term viability of these methods, it is important to prioritize the utilization of locally derived raw materials and to prioritize production on a smaller scale.

In spite of the numerous advantages that come with using conventional ways to extract oil, these techniques are not devoid of difficulties. In terms of restrictions, the scale of production is one of the most significant. The production of huge volumes of oil is made more difficult by the fact that traditional methods are frequently labor-intensive and time-consuming. Consequently, this has resulted in the widespread use of industrialized oil extraction techniques in a variety of regions across the globe. However, there is a growing movement toward recovering and preserving historic oil extraction processes, particularly in the context of sustainable agriculture and natural health. This effort is particularly important in maintaining natural health.

Over the past several years, there has been a rising awareness of the health benefits of natural, unprocessed oils, which has led to an increase in the demand for artisanal oils of high quality. Because of this, there has been a resurgence in interest in traditional methods of oil extraction, particularly in the manufacture of specialty oils such as extra-virgin olive oil, cold-pressed coconut oil, and unrefined sesame oil. These oils are frequently advertised as luxury products because of their excellent flavor, nutritional richness, and health benefits. All of these factors contribute to their high value.

Not only are oils that have been traditionally extracted valuable for their culinary and therapeutic applications, but they are also highly prized for their cosmetic qualities. As a result of their high levels of antioxidants and important fatty acids, many of the oils that are extracted using traditional methods, such as rosehip oil, argan oil, and jojoba oil, are widely used as components in natural skincare products. Because of the widespread belief that they are more effective than their processed equivalents, these oils are frequently utilized in their raw and unadulterated forms. The use of traditional oils in skincare has its origins in ancient beauty rituals, in which oils were applied to the skin in order to prevent damage and provide nourishment.

There is also a significant contribution that traditional oil extraction methods make to the conservation of biodiversity and the support of local economies. The traditional extraction of oil is carried out by small-scale farmers and craftspeople in many regions of the world. These individuals rely on these techniques for their means of subsistence (or livelihood). These communities are able to retain native plant species and preserve traditional knowledge that has been passed down from generation to generation because they continue to use traditional ways of oil production. This is of utmost significance in areas where the implementation of industrial agriculture and contemporary extraction techniques has resulted in the reduction of biodiversity and the deterioration of cultural assets.

As a conclusion, traditional methods of oil extraction provide a one-of-a-kind combination of history, culture, and environmental responsibility. Even if contemporary technology has completely revolutionized the process of oil production, traditional methods continue to be valuable because of their capacity to maintain the natural properties of the oil and to support production on a modest scale that is both sustainable and environmentally friendly. Whether they are utilized in the kitchen, cosmetics, medicine, or religious rites, oils that have been extracted by ancient methods are a demonstration of the profound link that exists between humans and the natural world. Traditional oil extraction techniques are likely to play an increasingly important role in the manufacture of high-quality, artisanal oils as the interest in natural health and sustainable living continues to develop across the globe. These techniques not only provide a window into the past, but they also offer a way forward for a more environmentally friendly and conscientious approach to the production of oil to be taken.

Cultural and Ritualistic Uses

As a reflection of the profound link that exists between humans and the natural world, oils have been utilized in a major manner throughout the course of human history in the context of cultural and ritualistic traditions. In a wide variety of communities, the process of extracting and making use of oils derived from plants, seeds, nuts, and other natural sources has been intricately entwined with spiritual, medical, and cultural traditions. Oils are more than just useful components for cooking or skin care in many different cultures; they are also considered sacred elements that are utilized to allow communion with the divine, promote healing, and signify purity and transformation. By gaining an understanding of these cultural and ritualistic applications, one can gain insight into the overall significance of oils throughout the course of human history, as well as their continued relevance in contemporary times.

The use of oils in cultural and ritual contexts can be traced back to ancient Egypt, which is one of the earliest documented uses of oils known to exist. Ancient Egyptians were among the first people to make use of essential oils, and they did so in a variety of contexts, including religious rituals and everyday life. During the embalming procedure, essential oils such as frankincense, myrrh, and cedarwood were utilized. During the process of preserving the bodies of the departed and ensuring that they had a peaceful transfer into the afterlife, these oils played an important role. Moreover, these oils, which were believed to possess characteristics of protection and purification, were applied in the practice of anointing the living, particularly monarchs and priests, in order to signify their divine status and spiritual power. This was done in order to show that they were divine and possessed spiritual power. During religious ceremonies, priests would burn essential oils in temples with the intention of bringing the gods into the presence of the people praying to them. The end effect of this would be the production of a holy environment that was characterized by the presence of fragrant smoke. The reverence that the Egyptians held for oils extended beyond the realm of religion and death and covered not only their religious practices but also their daily ceremony practices. A profound spiritual connection to the land and the divine was represented by the use of oils in a variety of applications, including for cosmetics, medicine, and even as sacrifices to deities.

Similar to this, oils played a significant part in the religious and cultural acts that were carried out in ancient Greece. In particular, olive oil was treasured due to the fact that it possessed characteristics that were both flexible and symbolic. The ancient Greeks utilized olive oil in a broad variety of ceremonies, ranging from religious offerings to sports competitions among athletes. The winners of the Olympic Games were crowned with olive wreaths and anointed with olive oil, which served as a symbol of both their physical dexterity and the divine favor they had received. For the same reason that it was considered to convey the essence of life and fertility, olive oil was also offered to the gods at sacred ceremonies. Furthermore, the divine connections of olive oil were further strengthened by the fact that the goddess Athena was credited with bestowing the olive tree upon humanity in Greek mythology. Not only did olive oil have religious importance, but it was also utilized as a material that was both protective and healing. Olive oil was prescribed by Greek physicians, notably Hippocrates, for the treatment of wounds, skin disorders, and digestive issues. This highlights the significance of olive oil in both cultural and therapeutic contexts.

Within the context of ancient Rome, the cultural and ritualistic application of oils was of comparable significance. The Romans, much like the Greeks, placed a high value on olive oil due to the spiritual and practical significance it possessed. To cleanse and moisturize the body, olive oil was used in Roman baths, which were an essential part of Roman culture. Olive oil was also used to clean the body. This ritual, which was considered to cleanse both the body and the mind, consisted of bathers rubbing oil into their bodies and then scraping it off using a device known as a strigil or strigil. Additionally, oils were utilized in religious rites, where they were presented to deities and deities of the gods and goddesses as a sign of commitment and appreciation. The anointing of leaders with oil was a symbol of their divine right to rule, and oil lamps were used to light temples and other sacred areas, which represented the enlightenment of the soul. Oil was utilized in Rome for a variety of purposes, including cooking, medicinal, and even used as a sort of currency in trade. Its cultural significance stretched to every aspect of daily life in Rome.

Not only was the Mediterranean region the only place in the ancient world where people used oils for religious and cultural purposes, but their use was widespread. According to the Ayurvedic system, which has been practiced in India for hundreds of years, the application of oils is deeply ingrained. To promote healing and spiritual equilibrium, the holistic medical practice known as Ayurveda places a strong emphasis on the utilization of oils. For instance, sesame oil is a significant component in a number of Ayurvedic treatments. This is due to the fact that it is said to possess characteristics that are both warming and grounding, which in turn promote both physical and emotional well-being. Oil massage, also known as "abhyanga," is a major practice in Ayurvedic rites. This practice involves applying oils to the body in order to bring the "doshas," or energies that are present inside the body, into harmony. It is thought that this exercise may cleanse the body of negative energy and restore equilibrium between the individual and the universe. This practice is not only medicinal, but it also has a profound spiritual significance. Additionally, oils are utilized in the performance of religious rites in Hinduism. One example of this is the burning of oil lamps during "puja" ceremonies, which is meant to represent the eradication of ignorance and the awakening of spiritual understanding.

Over the course of several centuries, oils have been utilized in a variety of cultural and ritualistic contexts throughout East Asia, particularly in China and Japan. For the purpose of treating various ailments, traditional Chinese medicine (TCM) makes use of oils that have been derived from various plants and herbs. These oils are considered to have special energetic characteristics that serve to balance the body's internal systems, hence promoting health and vitality. Essential oils such as camphor, tea tree, and ginger are often used in acupuncture and massage therapy to increase the energy flow, also known as "qi," that flows through the body. In Chinese rituals, oils have been employed to create a fragrant bridge between the spiritual and physical worlds. These oils have been used to honor ancestors and deities by contributing to the creation of incense and offerings. In a similar manner, the utilization of essential oils is profoundly intertwined with the practices of "Shinto" in Japan. Shinto is a form of spiritual cleansing that involves the utilization of aromatic oils and incense to cleanse the spirit and invite divine favors. As part of the Japanese practice known as "Kodo," which translates to "the art of appreciating incense," the ceremonial use of oils and scents is employed in order to encourage awareness and spiritual introspection.

Within the continent of Africa, the utilization of oils for cultural and ritualistic purposes is widespread, particularly within the context of indigenous activities and spiritual rituals. Palm oil, for instance, is utilized in religious ceremonies and sacrifices to deities and ancestors in West African countries. Anointing the body with palm oil, which is regarded as a sacred substance, is done during spiritual rites because it is thought to carry energy that is positive and beneficial to life. Palm oil is typically presented to the "orishas" or gods in Yoruba theology as part of the ritual sacrifices and prayers that are performed. Not only is shea butter, another oil that is Indigenous to West Africa, utilized in daily living but it is also utilized in spiritual rituals. The application of shea butter to the skin at rites of passage, such as childbirth and marriage, is a traditional practice that is meant to symbolize protection and blessings. These oils are prized not only for their physical properties but also for their spiritual importance, which represents the interconnectedness of life, nature, and the divine. Other reasons for their value include their physical properties.

Additionally, the indigenous cultures of the Americas make use of oils in a fashion that is both culturally significant and ritualistic. In their spiritual and healing traditions, unique American tribes have been using oils for a very long time. These oils are typically obtained from plants that are unique to their regions. Sage oil, which is produced from the sacred sage plant, is one example of a substance that is utilized in "smudging" ceremonies for the purpose of purifying individuals and environments from negative energy. Additionally, oils made from cedarwood and sweetgrass are utilized in purification rituals. It is claimed that the aromatic characteristics of these oils can establish a connection between the physical world and the spiritual sector. Not only are these oils utilized for their fragrance attributes, but they are also utilized for their profound symbolic value, which symbolizes the unification of several elements, including earth, air, fire, and water. Healing activities involve the application of oils to the body during prayers and chants in order to summon both spiritual and bodily healing. In addition to their use in purification, oils are also utilized in healing practices.

The Middle East has a long and illustrious history of incorporating the use of oils into cultural and ritualistic acts on a regular basis. Both frankincense and myrrh, which are considered to be two of the most cherished oils in the area, have been utilized in religious rites for thousands of years. In ancient Mesopotamia and the Arabian Peninsula, frankincense was burned as a gift to the gods. It was believed that the smoke from the burning of frankincense would carry prayers straight to the skies. Myrrh, which is well-known for its curative qualities, was utilized in the practice of burial ceremonies to anoint the bodies of the departed, so guaranteeing that they would have a smooth transition into the hereafter. These oils, which are described in holy scriptures such as the Bible and the Quran, continue to be very important to the spiritual practices of both the Christian religion and the Islamic religion. The anointing of the Holy Spirit is represented in Christian rites by the use of oils such as chrism, which is a blend of olive oil and balsam. These oils are used in sacraments such as baptism and confirmation. In Islamic tradition, oils such as rose and oud are utilized in the process of personal grooming as well as religious ceremonies. This serves to emphasize the significance of cleanliness and attractiveness in the process of spiritual development.

The use of oils in cultural and ritualistic contexts is not limited to ancient or indigenous activities; rather, it continues to flourish in contemporary spiritual practices. In current alternative therapeutic therapies, such as aromatherapy, oils are utilized to improve emotional and spiritual well-being. Aromatherapy is one popular example. It is claimed that essential oils, such as those derived from lavender, eucalyptus, and peppermint, have therapeutic characteristics that can help alleviate stress, improve meditation, and encourage spiritual development. There are a lot of modern spiritual practitioners who use oils as part of their daily rituals. They use them to anoint the body, purify their environment, or strengthen their connection to the divine. A newfound appreciation for the cultural and spiritual value of oils has emerged as a result of the rebirth of interest in natural health and well-being. This is especially true in the context of activities such as yoga, meditation, and energy healing.

The symbolic value of oils extends to the religious acts that are practiced in modern times as well. Olive oil, for instance, is used to light the menorah during the Hanukkah holiday in Judaism. This is done to commemorate the miracle of the oil that burnt for eight days in the Temple of Jerusalem. In the Christian religion, the use of oils in sacraments, such as the anointing of the sick and holy orders, continues to symbolize the presence of the divine and the recuperative power of faith. The use of oils in rites such as weddings, funerals, and personal milestones indicates the persistent belief in the symbolic and transforming effects of oils, even in circumstances that are not religious in nature.

Oils have the ability to bridge the gap between the physical and spiritual realms, and this has been the case throughout all civilizations and throughout history. Incorporating them into rituals and ceremonies demonstrates a profound reverence for the natural world as well as an awareness of the interdependence of all living things. In the cultural and spiritual rituals of humanity, oils retain a holy place not only for the purpose of anointing the body but also for the purpose of purifying spaces and honoring the divine. It is a testament to the enduring force of nature and the important role that oils play in the human search for meaning, healing, and connection that their relevance has persisted over long periods of time. An increasing number of people are becoming interested in natural and holistic practices, and it is likely that the cultural and ritualistic applications of oils will continue to be an essential component of both old traditions and contemporary spiritual journeys.

The many practices that surround the manufacture, processing, and use of oils are also illustrative of the profound reverence that exists for oils in a variety of different civilizations. Every culture has developed its own distinctive techniques for extracting and utilizing oils, which are a reflection of the local beliefs and the conditions of the environment. For example, in areas where particular plants are able to flourish in abundance, such as the Mediterranean region, the production of olive oil has become an essential component of both the culinary and spiritual lives of the people who live there. Olives are traditionally pressed using procedures that emphasize a reverence for the natural environment and an awareness of the significance of work in the process of making something sacred. These methods are often performed by hand.

In many different cultures, the process of extracting oil is considered to be an art form that is infused with ceremonial and ritualistic practices. In many cases, the spiritual value of the oils themselves is reflected in the painstaking processes used in the extraction process, the careful selection of raw materials, and the ceremonial features that surround the final product. It is possible that traditional activities in areas where coconut oil is widely available, for instance, involve community gatherings in which families get together to harvest oil from coconuts. During this procedure, singing or chanting is frequently performed, which serves to strengthen the social and spiritual ties that exist within the community. Similar to this, the creation of oils is a communal activity that is common in many indigenous cultures. This activity helps to develop a link to heritage and ancestors, which in turn ensures that the knowledge of traditional techniques is passed down from generation to generation.

Additionally, the utilization of oils in spiritual practices frequently extends beyond regional limits, with some oils obtaining universal importance as a result of the distinctive qualities that they possess. The calming and soothing qualities of lavender oil, for instance, have garnered widespread praise all around the world. For the purpose of promoting relaxation and fostering an atmosphere of serenity, it is utilized in meditation and prayer in a number of different cultures. Certain oils are able to adapt to a variety of cultural environments while still retaining their core properties because of their adaptability. In a similar vein, the utilization of essential oils such as peppermint and eucalyptus for the purpose of promoting respiratory health is a practice that is present in a number of different cultures, demonstrating a widespread knowledge of the curative qualities of the natural world.

It is becoming increasingly apparent that cultural behaviors about oil use are becoming more intertwined as the world continues to become more interconnected. A combination of ancient and contemporary methods that honor the efficacy of oils has emerged as a result of the proliferation of wellness movements around the world. People are increasingly interested in holistic approaches to health and well-being, which has led to the rise in popularity of aromatherapy, which blends oils associated with a variety of cultural traditions. The incorporation of many cultural viewpoints has resulted in an enhanced comprehension of the ways in which oils can be utilized for the purpose of emotional, bodily, and spiritual healing, hence rendering the advantages of these oils available to a more extensive audience.

There is a growing understanding of the cultural and spiritual value of oils, which is reflected in the rebirth of interest in natural medicines and sustainable practices. In order to show respect for the time-honored customs that have been in place for millennia, many modern practitioners highlight the significance of obtaining oils in a manner that is both ethical and environmentally responsible. The resurrection of artisanal production processes that are reflective of cultural heritage has been brought about as a result of the desire for natural oils of superior quality. In this environment, the production of oils is considered not only as a means of making cash but also as a way of preserving cultural identity and establishing communal relationships. In other words, both of these goals are accomplished simultaneously.

Oils, in addition to their practical applications, are frequently rich in symbolism and meaning within the context of cultural and spiritual frameworks. In rituals, the utilization of particular oils can be charged with significant meaning, acting as a medium through which spiritual connection and transformation might take place. For instance, in a number of different religious traditions, the act of anointing with oil is significant because it represents empowerment, healing, and protection. In Christian rituals, anointing oil is used to symbolize the presence of the Holy Spirit. On the other hand, in many African cultures, oils are used to symbolize blessings and protection from negative spirits. These symbolic elements bring to light the multifaceted character of oils, illuminating the fact that oils serve not only as physical objects but also as representations of more profound spiritual truths.

Furthermore, it is impossible to overstate the powerful emotional resonance that oils have in the context of cultural and ritualistic settings. There is a strong emotional connection that may be formed between individuals and their history through the fragrances and aromas that are connected with specific oils. These scents and aromas frequently prompt powerful recollections and feelings. Many individuals have said that the aroma of frankincense has the ability to cause them to be transported to hallowed places or to moments of great spiritual experience. In a similar vein, the scent of lavender may bring to mind a cherished member of the family who relied on it as a source of solace. It is via these sensory sensations that the concept that oils are not only products but rather carriers of cultural memory and emotional importance is presented and reinforced.

As an illustration of the enduring significance of these cultural and ceremonial applications, the incorporation of oils into everyday rituals and routines for the purpose of self-care is a contemporary spiritual practice that has become more popular. As a result of the oils' capacity to enhance one's awareness and foster a more profound connection with oneself, an increasing number of individuals are turning to them. The practice of diffusing essential oils during meditation or applying them during yoga sessions is a reflection of the growing knowledge of the interplay that exists between aroma, feeling, and spirituality. This awareness is represented in the practice of using essential oils during yoga sessions. This contemporary approach is consistent with traditional practices, which exemplify the lasting character of oils as instruments for the aim of facilitating personal growth and transformation.

At the same time, as we are conducting research on the application of oils in cultural and ritualistic contexts, it is of the utmost importance to acknowledge the necessity of interacting with these traditions in a respectful manner. In particular, the wellness industry is becoming increasingly marketed, which raises ethical questions about the appropriation of indigenous knowledge and the exploitation of cultural practices. Traditional oils are becoming increasingly commercialized. When it comes to the utilization of oil, various communities have developed long-standing customs that have been handed down from one generation to successive generations. If these customs are adopted or commercialized without the necessary degree of understanding or respect, it has the potential to result in a watering down of their significance and meaning. This could happen if the appropriate level of either understanding or respect is not present. The importance of recognizing the value of traditional knowledge and the significance of knowing the cultural context from which these practices originate cannot be understated. Both of these things are necessary. Having cultural knowledge when approaching these practices is something that is absolutely necessary for both customers and practitioners.

It is possible to draw the conclusion that the cultural and ritualistic applications of oils are a demonstration of the everlasting connection that exists between people and the natural world. Throughout the course of human history, oils have been utilized as potent symbols of connection, healing, and transformation. These symbols can be found in the spiritual rituals of ancient civilizations as well as in contemporary spiritual practices. There are a wide variety of applications that oils have to offer throughout a variety of civilizations, which is a reflection of the multifaceted nature of oils as both utilitarian substances and sacred elements. As we continue to navigate a world that is undergoing rapid development, the wisdom that is ingrained in these cultural traditions serves as a reminder to us that it is crucial to respect our relationships with the natural world and the spiritual components of our lives. This is especially important as we continue to navigate this fast-changing world. If we accept the many diverse traditions that surround oils and the complex tapestry of traditions that surround them, we may be able to generate a richer knowledge of ourselves, our communities, and our role for ourselves within the natural environment. Because of the power of oils, both in terms of the physical properties they possess and the cultural significance they hold, we are encouraged to dig into the profound depths of the human experience. These oils provide us with pathways to healing, connection, and spiritual awareness, and they do it in a significant way.

CHAPTER II

The Science of Essential Oils

Chemical Components

In the process of deciding the quality, applications, and effects of oils, the chemical components of oils are significant aspects that play a large role in having a significant influence. Oils are complex mixtures that contain a wide range of chemical constituents, and this is true regardless of whether they are derived from plants, seeds, or fruits. These compounds consist of fatty acids, triglycerides, essential oils, and several other chemicals that have a bioactive effect. Because of this, it is feasible to have a greater grasp of how oils act in the context of culinary applications, cosmetic formulations, and therapeutic treatments once their chemical components have been comprehended. Each type of oil has its own unique composition of chemical components, which defines its flavor, scent, and stability, as well as the health benefits it provides by affecting these properties. The vast majority of oils are made up of fatty acids, which are carboxylic acids that have an extended chain of hydrocarbons. Fatty acids are the fundamental components of oils.

Saturated, monounsaturated, and polyunsaturated fatty acids are the three primary categories that can be used to classify these chemical compounds. All saturated fatty acids, including palmitic and stearic acids, are in a solid state at normal temperature because they do not contain any double bonds between the carbon atoms that make up their structure. They are frequently discovered in oils such as coconut oil and palm oil, which are highly valued for their consistency and extend the amount of time they can be stored. At room temperature, monounsaturated fatty acids, such as oleic acid, which can be found in olive oil, are typically liquid. Monounsaturated fatty acids often have one double bond. Multiple double bonds are present in polyunsaturated fatty acids, which can be found in oils such as flaxseed oil and sunflower oil. Linoleic and alpha-linolenic acids are examples of polyunsaturated fatty acids. These fatty acids are necessary for human health because the body is unable to produce them on its own and must instead receive them from the consumption of different foods.

The nutritional profile of oil and the health advantages it offers are substantially influenced by the proportion of fatty acids that it contains. For instance, oils that are high in monounsaturated fats, such as olive oil, have been linked to favorable effects on cardiovascular health, including the reduction of inflammation and the enhancement of cholesterol levels. On the other hand, when consumed in excessive amounts, oils that are high in saturated fats may be associated with negative consequences on one's health. Due to this, there has been an increase in the demand for oils that have fat profiles that are more beneficial to one's health, with a particular emphasis on polyunsaturated fats, specifically omega-3 and omega-6 fatty acids. The function of the brain, the health of the cardiovascular system, and overall well-being are all significantly impacted by these critical fatty acids.

Triglycerides are esters that are generated from glycerol and three different fatty acids. Triglycerides are found in oils also, in addition to fatty acids. Triglycerides are the most common type of fat that is stored in the body, and they are also a large component of fats that are consumed through food. There is a wide range of triglyceride compositions found in oils, which has an impact on the physical qualities and applications of these oils. As an illustration, oils that contain a high concentration of unsaturated triglycerides have a tendency to retain their liquid state at room temperature, which makes them excellent for use as salad dressings and cooking oils. On the other hand, oils that have a higher percentage of saturated triglycerides are more solid, which is why they are popular for use in baking and frying.

One further key component of oils is the existence of essential oils, which are chemicals that are volatile and add to the scent and flavor of the oil. There are many different components of plants that can be used to extract essential oils, such as the leaves, flowers, bark, and fruits. The aromas that are typical of many oils, such as the sweet aroma of lavender oil or the refreshing scent of peppermint oil, are a result of their presence. Due to the therapeutic effects that these aromatic compounds possess, they are frequently utilized in aromatherapy, fragrances, and natural health products. Terpenes, aldehydes, alcohols, esters, and phenols are just a few of the chemical elements that can be found in essential oils. Each of these constituents contributes a different set of benefits to the essential oil.

Terpenes, for example, are representative of a huge and varied category of organic chemicals that are produced by a wide variety of plant species. They have been investigated for the possible therapeutic effects that they may have, and they are responsible for the characteristic aromas that are associated with a variety of essential oils. For instance, limonene, which is included in citrus oils, has been demonstrated to possess anti-inflammatory and mood-enhancing qualities. Other types of terpenes, such as pinene and linalool, are well-known for their capacity to induce a state of relaxation and reduce feelings of anxiety. Terpenes are present in essential oils, and their presence not only contributes to the health benefits of essential oils but also enriches the sensory experience of utilizing essential oils.

Oils can also contain a variety of bioactive chemicals, such as antioxidants, vitamins, and phytosterols, as part of their chemical composition. In order to prevent oxidative deterioration, which can result in rancidity and the production of damaging free radicals, antioxidants are an essential component in the oil's defense against oxidative degradation. Additionally, oils that are abundant in antioxidants, such as vitamin E, have the ability to extend the shelf life of the oil and offer extra health benefits. The capacity of vitamin E to protect and revitalize the skin is one of the reasons why it is frequently incorporated in cosmetic formulations. Vitamin E is well-known for its nourishing effects that are beneficial to the skin.

In addition, phytosterols are an essential component of a wide variety of oils. The molecular structure of these chemicals originating from plants is comparable to that of cholesterol, and they have the potential to assist in lowering cholesterol levels in the body. They are especially prevalent in oils such as olive and sunflower oil, and they are known for the function that they play in promoting the health of the heart. Other bioactive substances, in addition to the presence of phytosterols, are responsible for the delicious and aromatic qualities of some oils, as well as the nutritional benefits they provide.

It is possible for the extraction procedure that is used to acquire oils to have a considerable impact on the chemical composition of the oils. Cold pressing and expeller pressing are two examples of traditional extraction techniques that have a tendency to maintain the natural components of the oil in their original state. As a result of the fact that these techniques preserve the flavor, aroma, and nutritional profile of the oil, they are highly regarded in culinary and therapeutic applications. On the other hand, industrial extraction techniques, such as solvent extraction or refining, have the potential to remove some of the oil's beneficial components and alter its qualities. As a result, there has been an increase in the demand for oils that have undergone little processing, therefore preserving their natural properties and offering the greatest possible health advantages.

The conditions under which oils are stored, the amount of light they are exposed to, and the temperature can all have an impact on the integrity of the oils. Because oils are sensitive to oxidation, rancidity, as well as a reduction in flavor and nutritional value, can occur as a result of this process. For the purpose of preserving the chemical integrity of oils, it is imperative that they be stored in containers that are dark, airtight, and away from temperature sources. When it comes to maximizing the benefits of oils in their culinary, cosmetic, and therapeutic applications, it is essential for both consumers and producers to have a thorough understanding of these elements.

Furthermore, the interplay of chemical components within oils can result in synergistic effects, which boost the overall advantages of the oils. An example of this would be the combination of fatty acids, essential oils, and antioxidants, which can result in enhanced anti-inflammatory, antibacterial, and antioxidant capabilities. Additionally, this synergy is most noticeable in oils that are utilized in traditional medicine systems. In these systems, precise combinations of oils are produced to treat a variety of health concerns. The holistic method of using oils acknowledges the interconnection of the chemical components that make up oils as well as the collective impact that these components have on one's health.

The therapeutic properties of essential oils are utilized in the field of aromatherapy, which involves the utilization of the chemical components of essential oils. Essential oils have been demonstrated to have a variety of effects on the body and mind, each of which is distinct from the others according to the chemical components that they contain. As an illustration, oils that are rich in sesquiterpenes, such as sandalwood, are thought to encourage relaxation and grounding, which makes them an excellent choice for meditation techniques. On the other hand, oils that are high in phenols, such as those found in oregano and thyme, have powerful antibacterial capabilities, which makes them useful in natural health applications.

As a result of the oil's position in contemporary wellness practices, there has been a rebirth of interest in the chemical components of oils as well as the possible benefits they may offer. A significant increase in the demand for high-quality oils can be attributed to the fact that customers are looking for natural alternatives to manufactured items. As a result of this tendency, there has been a rise in research about the chemical profiles of different oils, which has led to the discovery of new insights into the qualities and applications of these oils. Numerous traditional uses of oils have been validated by scientific research, establishing their position as an integral part of modern wellness treatments.

In addition to the positive effects that oils have on one's health, the chemical components of oils also have an effect on the sensory aspects of oils, which is why oils are so important to the culinary arts and cuisine. It is the existence of particular volatile compounds that determines the flavor profiles of oils. These compounds can have a wide variety of flavors, ranging from earthy and nutty to flowery and fruity. As an illustration, the high quantities of oleocanthal that are present in extra virgin olive oil are responsible for the oil's opulent and peppery flavor. Oleocanthal is a chemical that has both flavor and health benefits. When it comes to their culinary creations, both professional chefs and home cooks are able to make more educated decisions when they have a thorough understanding of the chemical components that contribute to the flavor of oils.

Additionally, oils have applications in the cosmetics and personal care items that are available, which further demonstrates their versatility. The emollient characteristics, absorption rates, and overall efficiency of oils in skin care formulations are all influenced by the chemical composition of the oils. Products that have a high concentration of essential fatty acids, such as argan oil and jojoba oil, are highly valued for their capacity to hydrate and nourish the skin. Because of the presence of antioxidants and vitamins in these oils, their effectiveness is further enhanced, which is why they are frequently used in treatments that are intended to moisturize and prevent the aging process.

For the purpose of comprehending the numerous characteristics, applications, and benefits that oils contain, it is vital to have a fundamental understanding of the chemical components that oils are composed of. Fatty acids, triglycerides, essential oils, and bioactive compounds are only a few of the components that play a significant role in determining the quality of oils due to their individual contributions. Bioactive compounds are also included among the other components. The extraction methods that are used, the circumstances under which the oils are stored, and the interactions that take place between the chemical ingredients are all additional aspects that have an impact on the quality and effectiveness of oils. In spite of the fact that there is a growing interest in natural health, wellness, and culinary arts, the analysis of the chemical components of oils continues to be an area that is actively being researched. Through this work, we have gained a better understanding of the enormous impact that these ancient compounds have on each of our lives. Deciphering the mysteries of oils allows us to build a more profound awareness of their power, versatility, and ability to improve our well-being in a range of aspects of life. This insight can be gained by deciphering the mysteries of oils.

This complex tapestry of oils continues to emerge as a result of continual research and discovery, which reveals new ideas and uses that honor the incredible chemistry that nature possesses.

How Oils Affect the Body

There is a significant impact that oils, both essential and nutritional, have on the human body. These oils have an effect on a wide variety of physiological processes, which in turn can improve general health and well-being. Through an understanding of their chemical compositions, the function that oils play in nutrition, and the ways in which they are utilized in both conventional and alternative medicine, one can gain an understanding of the impact that oils have on the body. Examining the nutritional characteristics of oils, as well as their therapeutic applications and the effects they have on both physical and mental health, is a part of the investigation into how oils influence the physique.

Olive oil, coconut oil, and avocado oil are examples of dietary oils that are predominantly constituted of fatty acids. Fatty acids are necessary for a wide variety of vital body functions. These fatty acids can be classified into three distinct categories: saturated, monounsaturated, and polyunsaturated. Each of these types has a unique role in the body's metabolism and on the body's overall health. Due to the fact that they are linked to elevated cholesterol levels and cardiovascular illness, saturated fats, which are frequently present in animal products and certain plant oils, have been regarded with apprehension for a considerable amount of time. The influence of saturated fats, on the other hand, may be contingent on the source of the fat as well as the general context of the diet, according to a recent study. As an example, coconut oil, which is abundant in medium-chain triglycerides (MCTs), may offer a variety of health advantages, such as enhanced energy metabolism and the possibility of affecting weight management.

Monounsaturated fats, which are found in abundance in oils such as olive oil, are well acknowledged for their beneficial effects on cardiovascular health. In order to lessen the risk of cardiovascular disorders, these fats can help reduce levels of bad cholesterol (LDL) while simultaneously boosting levels of good cholesterol (HDL). One of the many health benefits that have been linked to the Mediterranean diet, which places a strong emphasis on the intake of olive oil, is a decreased risk of developing cardiovascular disease, stroke, and even certain types of cancer. Olive oil contains a number of antioxidants, including polyphenols, which play an important part in the fight against oxidative stress. This helps to further protect the body from developing chronic diseases.

Polyunsaturated fats, which typically consist of omega-3 and omega-6 fatty acids, are absolutely necessary for achieving and sustaining the highest possible level of health. As a result of the fact that the body is unable to produce certain fatty acids on its own, they are referred to as "essential" fatty acids. Known for their anti-inflammatory effects and importance in maintaining brain health, omega-3 fatty acids can be found in a variety of foods, including flaxseed oil, fish oil, and walnuts. Omega-3 fatty acids have been found to improve cognitive performance, alleviate symptoms of anxiety and sadness, and even lessen the risk of neurodegenerative illnesses, according to research with a scientific basis. Additionally, these fats are an essential component of the formation of cell membranes and play an important part in the generation of hormones, the transmission of signals between cells, and the overall metabolic processes.

Omega-6 fatty acids, on the other hand, which may be found in oils like sunflower and corn oil, are also responsible for several important functions within the body. On the other hand, the ordinary diet of Westerners frequently contains an excessive amount of omega-6 fatty acids, which can result in an imbalance that may contribute to inflammation and other health problems. The ratio of omega-3 to omega-6 fatty acids needs to be brought into better balance in order to achieve maximum health. The consumption of oils that are abundant in omega-3 fatty acids can help reduce the inflammatory effects that are caused by an excessive intake of omega-6 fatty acids, hence contributing to improved general health.

Oils have the potential to be used for medicinal purposes that go beyond their nutritional component. It is possible for essential oils, which are obtained from a wide variety of plants, to have distinctive chemical compositions that can have significant effects on both the body and the mind. These volatile compounds are utilized in aromatherapy, massage, and topical applications, which allows for the utilization of their benefits for the purpose of achieving both physical and mental healing. Essential oils, such as lavender or eucalyptus, can be inhaled to produce a variety of effects, including relaxation and the alleviation of stress, as well as improvements in respiratory function and an improvement in mood. Inhaled compounds interact with the limbic system of the brain, which in turn influences emotions, memory, and physiological reactions. However, the olfactory system plays a significant part in the way that these oils affect the body.

Additionally, essential oils that are administered topically might have an effect on the body. By penetrating the dermal layers of the skin and entering the bloodstream, essential oils are able to exert therapeutic effects on a variety of organs and systems when they are applied to the skin. It is common practice to use tea tree oil as a treatment for skin disorders such as acne and fungal infections. Tea tree oil is well-known for its antibacterial capabilities. As a result of their ability to alleviate muscle aches and respiratory difficulties, oils such as peppermint and eucalyptus are frequently used. These oils provide a cooling and calming impact. On the other hand, it is of the utmost importance to make sure that essential oils are utilized correctly, as some of them might cause allergic responses or skin irritation if they are used without being diluted. It is common practice to use carrier oils, such as jojoba or almond oil, to lower the concentration of essential oils in order to ensure their safe use.

Certain oils, particularly those derived from cannabis, such as hemp seed oil and CBD oil, are known to interact with the endocannabinoid system (ECS) of the nervous system. In addition to regulating a variety of physiological processes, such as pain, inflammation, and mood, the endocannabinoid system (ECS) is a complex network of receptors and agents. Due to the fact that the cannabinoids that are present in hemp oil interact with the endocannabinoid system (ECS), it has the ability to alleviate chronic pain, anxiety, and more. With promising results in a variety of areas, including the management of epilepsy, the reduction of anxiety, and the effects of anti-inflammatory agents, research into the therapeutic applications of cannabis oils continues to expand.

There is also a significant role that oils play in the health of the skin. This protective function of the skin can be enhanced by the use of oils, which act as a barrier to protect the body from the elements of the environment. In addition to restoring the skin's moisture barrier, improving elasticity, and reducing the appearance of fine lines and wrinkles, oils that are rich in fatty acids, such as rosehip oil and argan oil, can also help. To add insult to injury, the antioxidant properties of particular oils shield the skin from the damaging effects of oxidative stress and prevent premature aging processes. When used in conjunction with skincare routines, oils have the potential to result in skin that is both healthier and more radiant.

The influence of oils on the body is not restricted to the realm of physical health; they can also have an effect on the mental well-being of the individual. Oils and essential oils, in particular, can elicit emotional responses and have an effect on mood through the sensory experiences that they provide. Citrus oils, such as bergamot and lemon, for instance, are well-known for helping to alleviate symptoms of depression and anxiety due to their uplifting properties. Numerous studies have been conducted on the calming effects of lavender oil, and the findings of these studies have demonstrated that lavender oil is effective in lowering stress levels, fostering relaxation, and enhancing the quality of sleep. It has become increasingly popular as a complementary therapy for mental health conditions to use aromatherapy, which involves the inhalation of essential oils as well as their application topically.

It is also reflected in the practices of traditional medicine that oils have a relationship with the body. Throughout the centuries, numerous cultures all over the world have made use of oils because they have recognized the potential benefits that oils can provide for health and healing. Essential oils, such as sesame oil, are utilized in Ayurvedic medicine for a variety of therapeutic purposes, including massage and detoxification, among others. Traditional Chinese Medicine (TCM) makes use of oils and herbal infusions due to the fact that they have the ability to promote harmony within the body and balance the body. Oils play a multidimensional function in supporting well-being, which is highlighted by these holistic approaches to health, which emphasize the interdependence of the body, mind, and spirit.

One further significant feature of the oil's influence on the body is the fact that it is used in cooking. The addition of culinary oils to dishes not only imparts flavor but also supplies the body with vital elements that are beneficial to health. There is a correlation between the type of oil used in cooking and the nutritional composition of the food that is being prepared. With olive oil, for instance, the absorption of fat-soluble vitamins (A, D, E, and K) from vegetables can be improved, resulting in a meal that is higher in nutrient density. Olive oil can also be used as a cooking fat. It is important to note that the stability and health qualities of oils can be influenced by the cooking method as well as the temperature. There are certain oils, such as extra virgin olive oil, that have a relatively high smoke point, which makes them acceptable for a variety of cooking methods. On the other hand, flaxseed oil is best utilized without being cooked in order to maintain its nutritional benefits over time.

In recent years, there has been a renaissance of interest in the culinary and therapeutic applications of oils, which can be attributed to the increased understanding of the health advantages. There has been a shift toward oils that are minimally processed and high in bioactive components as a result of consumers being more health conscious and looking for natural alternatives to synthetic products. With an increased focus on quality and sourcing, this movement has led to a more comprehensive understanding of the function that oils play in nutrition, health, and wellness.

In addition, the effects of oils on the body might be affected by individual factors, including as genetics, lifestyle, and preexisting health disorders like asthma and diabetes. A growing number of people are turning to personalized nutrition, which takes into account these aspects, as a means of improving their health through the choices they make regarding their food and lifestyle. Consuming dietary oils that are specifically developed to satisfy the health goals of those who have certain health concerns, such as high cholesterol or inflammation, could be beneficial for those individuals who have already established their health goals. One can take a more tailored approach to nutrition and wellness if they are aware of the personal impacts that different oils have on the body. This is because different oils have different effects on different people.

As researchers continue to delve further into the complex relationships that exist between oils and health, the future of oil research holds a plethora of exciting possibilities. Extensive research is currently being conducted with the objective of clarifying the mechanisms via which oils exert their effects on the body. This is being done in order to shed light on the potential medicinal applications of oils. This research may lead to the development of new dietary guidelines, the creation of one-of-a-kind medicinal products, and the introduction of novel applications of oils in a range of contexts that are related to health and wellness.

As a consequence of this, oils have a significant influence on the body, which includes a wide range of physiological processes as well as the outcomes of many health disorders. There is a wide variety of major repercussions that may be attributed to various kinds of oils, such as essential oils used for therapeutic purposes and dietary oils that are rich in vital fatty acids. As a result of having an awareness of the chemical compositions, nutritional properties, and medical applications of oils, it is possible to acquire valuable insights into the functions that oils play in supporting health and well-being. As more and more information about oils becomes available, one of the most important areas of research that will continue to be conducted is the power of oils to improve both physical and mental health. This will assist folks in making decisions that are healthier and in adopting lifestyles that are healthier. By adopting a holistic approach to health that recognizes the inherent power of oils, individuals are able to unlock the mysteries of nature and harness the advantages of these ancient substances for contemporary living. This is made possible by the implementation of a holistic approach to health.

Research and Modern Validation

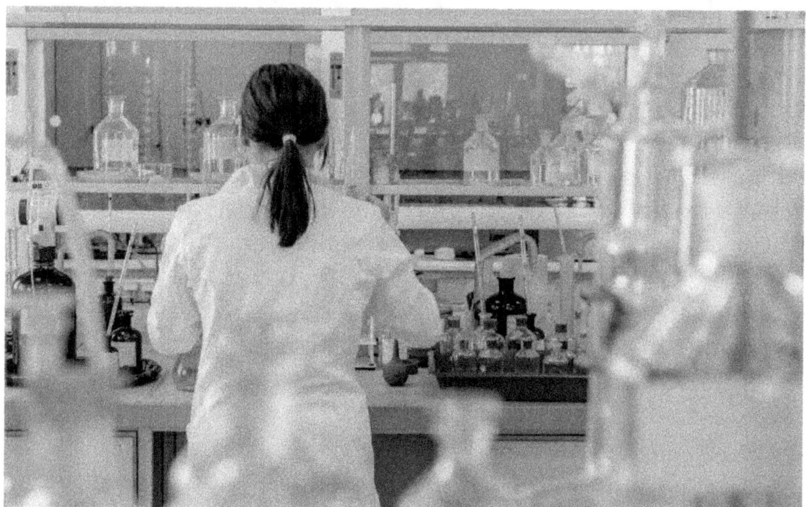

With a growing interest in natural therapies, alternative medicine, and the integration of traditional knowledge with modern scientific methodologies, research into the efficacy and applications of oils has gained substantial impetus in recent decades. This is primarily motivated by the fact that there has been a renewed interest in each of these areas. Numerous long-held ideas on the medicinal benefits of oils have been validated as a result of this boom in research, which has also revealed fresh insights into the pathways upon which oils exert their effects. In order to investigate the biological effects that essential oils, plant-based carrier oils, and dietary oils have on health, illness prevention, and overall well-being, comprehensive research is being conducted on all three types of oils. Researchers who are interested in understanding how oils function and how they might be effectively incorporated into modern health and wellness practices have both obstacles and opportunities due to the complexity of oils, which includes their multifaceted chemical compositions and the ways in which they interact with the human body.

Oils have been utilized throughout history for a variety of purposes, including culinary, medical, and spiritual applications. Throughout history, civilizations such as the Egyptians, Greeks, and Romans have included oils in rituals, healing practices, and personal care routines, among other things. The continuous usage of oils in present times can be traced back to the historical significance certain oils have held throughout history. However, given the stringent requirements of contemporary scientific research, the empirical evidence that was based on observation and conventional knowledge was not sufficient to meet the requirements. This is where research, which has its roots in clinical trials, biochemical analysis, and randomized controlled studies, has been essential in providing evidence-based validation for the use of oils in the treatment of diseases, the enhancement of mental health, and the promotion of total physical wellness.

The examination of essential oils, which are molecules that are volatile and fragrant and are extracted from various parts of plants such as leaves, flowers, stems, and roots, was a crucial step in the establishment of the current scientific validation of oils. Essential oils have been the topic of research due to the potential antibacterial, anti-inflammatory, and antioxidant characteristics that they possess. It is possible that lavender oil is one of the essential oils that has been studied the most, particularly in relation to the alleviation of stress and anxiety, as well as the enhancement of sleep capacity. The inhalation of lavender essential oil has been shown in a number of studies to be effective in lowering anxiety levels in individuals who are undergoing stressful medical procedures, such as dental treatments or surgical procedures. There is a connection between the calming effects of lavender and its interaction with the limbic system of the brain, which is an important part of the neurological system and plays a significant role in the regulation of emotions. Furthermore, additional research has demonstrated that lavender has the potential to enhance the quality of sleep, particularly in persons who are afflicted with insomnia, by fostering relaxation and lowering restlessness. According to the findings of this study, the traditional application of lavender in aromatherapy, where it has been utilized for generations to promote peace and well-being, has been validated.

There has been a significant amount of research conducted on peppermint oil because of its potential to heal a wide variety of common problems, ranging from digestive disorders to headaches. The use of peppermint oil as a treatment for irritable bowel syndrome (IBS) is one area of contemporary study that has garnered a lot of attention in recent years. It has been demonstrated through clinical trials that the consumption of peppermint oil in enteric-coated capsules can alleviate symptoms of irritable bowel syndrome (IBS) in individuals. These symptoms include stomach pain, bloating, and diarrhea. Menthol, the principal active component of the oil, possesses antispasmodic qualities, which means that it has the ability to relax the smooth muscles of the gastrointestinal tract, reducing discomfort and facilitating digestion. Peppermint oil has also been shown to be effective as a topical treatment for tension headaches, according to a study. Peppermint oil has been shown to diminish the severity of headaches when applied to the forehead and temples. This is due to the oil's capacity to enhance blood flow to the affected areas as well as its cooling effect. These studies not only corroborate the traditional use of peppermint oil but also shed light on the oil's potential to serve as a natural substitute for pharmaceuticals that are available without a prescription.

Another essential oil that has been shown to be useful in treating respiratory disorders is eucalyptus oil, which has been validated by scientific research. Within the realm of traditional medicine, eucalyptus has been utilized for a considerable amount of time to treat the symptoms of colds, coughs, and sinus congestion. Eucalyptol, a crucial ingredient present in eucalyptus oil, has been shown to possess powerful anti-inflammatory and mucolytic capabilities, which enables it to effectively release mucus and reduce inflammation in the respiratory system. This has been supported by a recent study. Eucalyptus oil is frequently utilized in the practice of steam inhalation and chest rubs for the purpose of alleviating congestion and enhancing breathing. It has been demonstrated through a number of clinical experiments that eucalyptol has the ability to enhance lung function and alleviate symptoms in those who suffer from chronic obstructive pulmonary disease (COPD) and asthma. This provides contemporary validation for the traditional application of eucalyptol in respiratory therapy.

Essential oils have also been the subject of a significant amount of research in recent times due to their antibacterial capabilities. Tea tree oil, in particular, has attracted a lot of attention due to the fact that it possesses antibacterial, antifungal, and antiviral properties that are broad-spectrum. Tea tree oil, which is indigenous to Australia, has been utilized by indigenous peoples for the treatment of skin diseases, wounds, and respiratory problems for hundreds of years. Tea tree oil has been shown to be effective against a wide range of pathogens, including Staphylococcus aureus, which is the bacteria that causes staph infections, and Candida albicans, which is the fungus that causes yeast infections. These findings have been derived from contemporary scientific research. The most important active component of the oil is terpinene-4-ol, which is thought to cause the cell membranes of fungi and bacteria to become disrupted, resulting in the death of the organisms. This research has led to the widespread usage of tea tree oil in commercial skincare products for the treatment of a variety of skin disorders, including acne, fungal infections, and other skin conditions. Its antibacterial characteristics have also made it a popular ingredient in natural household cleaning solutions, which further validates the traditional functions that it has been traditionally employed for.

Although essential oils have been the focus of a significant amount of research, dietary oils like olive oil, coconut oil, and fish oil have also been the topic of intensive investigation due to the many health advantages they offer. Olive oil, which is a fundamental component of the Mediterranean diet, has been the subject of a great deal of research dealing with cardiovascular health. It has been demonstrated through research that olive oil, and more specifically extra virgin olive oil, contains a high concentration of monounsaturated fats and polyphenols, both of which possess anti-inflammatory and antioxidant effects. Furthermore, these substances contribute to the reduction of oxidative stress and the reduction of levels of LDL cholesterol, which is usually referred to as "bad" cholesterol and is a factor in the development of cardiovascular disease. It has been demonstrated via extensive epidemiological research, such as the PREDIMED experiment, that consuming a diet that is abundant in olive oil is linked to a lower risk of cardiovascular disease, stroke, and mortality from any cause. Olive oil's reputation as one of the healthiest dietary oils has been strengthened as a result of this research, which validates its consumption for the purpose of enhancing heart health. Olive oil has been an essential component of Mediterranean diets for millennia.

In contemporary studies, coconut oil, which is another popular dietary oil, has been the subject of both acclaim and debate. In tropical countries, coconut oil has traditionally been utilized for a variety of purposes, including cooking, cosmetics, and hair treatment. It is abundant in medium-chain triglycerides (MCTs), which are thought to be digested differently than long-chain fats and may offer potential advantages for the management of weight as well as the production of energy. While some research has suggested that the medium-chain triglycerides (MCTs) found in coconut oil can boost metabolism and encourage fat burning, other studies have expressed concern about the high quantities of saturated fat found in coconut oil, which may cause an increase in cholesterol levels and contribute to the development of heart disease. As research into coconut oil continues, it continues to be a matter of discussion among health professionals. This serves to illustrate the complexity involved in authenticating traditional methods within the context of contemporary scientific standards.

Numerous studies have been conducted on fish oil, which is abundant in omega-3 fatty acids, to investigate its anti-inflammatory qualities as well as its role in supporting the health of the brain and the heart. It has been demonstrated that omega-3 fatty acids, in particular, eicosapentaenoic acid (EPA) and docosahexaenoic acid (DHA), can reduce inflammation, lower triglyceride levels, and improve the general health of the cardiovascular system. Supplements containing fish oil are frequently advised for people who have excessive cholesterol, high blood pressure, and other risk factors for cardiovascular disease. In addition, studies have shown that omega-3 fatty acids play a significant part in maintaining the health of the brain. Furthermore, research has shown that taking fish oil supplements may improve cognitive performance and lower the chance of developing neurodegenerative disorders like Alzheimer's. This contemporary affirmation of the health advantages of fish oil is in line with the traditional intake of fish in diets all over the world, particularly in coastal regions where seafood is a mainstay in the diet.

The practice of aromatherapy, which involves the application of essential oils for medicinal purposes, has also been a subject of research in recent times. The practice of aromatherapy has been utilized for a long time to facilitate relaxation, alleviate tension, and improve mental well-being. Recent research has demonstrated that inhaling specific essential oils, such as bergamot, ylang-ylang, and frankincense, can reduce levels of stress and anxiety by exerting an influence on the limbic system, which is responsible for regulating emotions and memory. For instance, it has been demonstrated that bergamot oil can reduce levels of cortisol, which is a hormone that is related to stress. On the other hand, frankincense oil has been discovered to increase emotions of peace and relaxation. The traditional use of aromatherapy to alleviate stress and improve mental health is given scientific legitimacy by these studies, which provide evidence for why aromatherapy is effective. Despite the expanding quantity of evidence that substantiates the advantages of oils, it is essential to keep in mind that not all oils are beneficial.

CHAPTER III

Physical Health Benefits

Treating Common Ailments

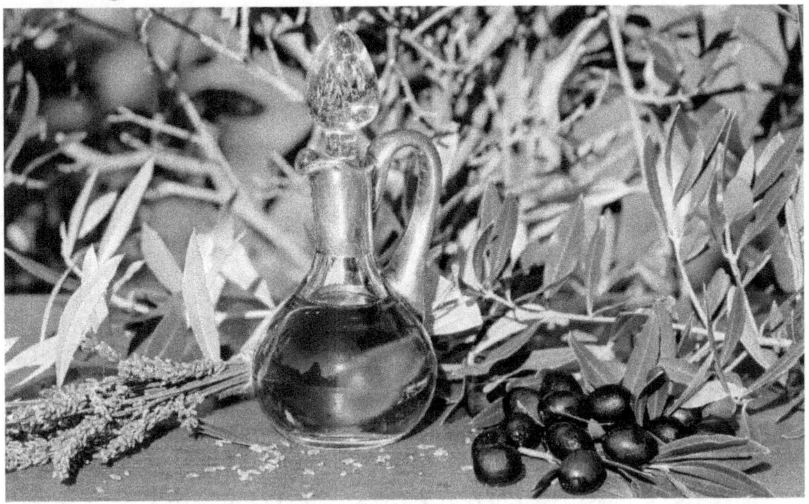

It is deeply established in human history to use oils for the treatment of common ailments. These oils have their origins in traditional medicine, cultural traditions, and treatments that have been around for centuries. Since ancient times, people have held oils, particularly those that are produced from plants, in high regard due to their curative qualities and their capacity to ease a wide range of physical and emotional ailments. Across a wide range of cultures and time periods, and regardless of whether they are administered physically, consumed, or inhaled through aromatherapy, oils have been utilized to a large degree in the treatment of many maladies. Oils have been brought back into the spotlight in recent decades as a result of the resurrection of natural therapies and holistic care. Additionally, the scientific community has shown a rising interest in confirming the effectiveness of oils in treating a wide variety of common health conditions.

When it comes to the treatment of respiratory problems, including colds, coughs, and sinus infections, one of the most common applications of oils is in the management of these conditions. In the past, essential oils such as eucalyptus, peppermint, and tea tree oil have been utilized widely for the treatment of diseases of this nature. For example, eucalyptus oil includes eucalyptol, a chemical that is well-known for its anti-inflammatory and mucolytic characteristics. These features assist in clearing airways and relieving congestion while also reducing inflammation. Inhaling eucalyptus oil through steam has been a tried-and-true treatment for bronchitis and colds for a very long time. It has been utilized for its menthol content, which not only helps to reduce congestion but also soothes sore throats and encourages better breathing. Peppermint oil, which is another potent essential oil, has been used for this purpose. The administration of peppermint oil topically or through inhalation is thought to activate the respiratory system, so offering relief from sinus pressure and congestion. Additionally, tea tree oil, which is well-known for its antibacterial characteristics, has been utilized in the treatment of infections that are associated with respiratory conditions, such as sinus infections caused by bacteria or fungi. Essential oils have been a staple for respiratory health for a number of reasons, including the fact that they provide a synthetic drug alternative that is both natural and effective.

Another region that has been shown to benefit from the application of oils in the treatment of common diseases is the digestive tract. In particular, peppermint oil has been the subject of a significant amount of research due to the favorable benefits it has on gastrointestinal disorders, particularly irritable bowel syndrome (IBS). Because of its antispasmodic qualities, it also helps to relax the muscles of the digestive tract, which in turn reduces symptoms such as stomach pain, bloating, and gas. For the purpose of alleviating symptoms of irritable bowel syndrome (IBS), peppermint oil capsules that have been coated to release the oil in the intestines rather than the stomach have demonstrated encouraging benefits in clinical trials. Ginger oil is another essential oil that is commonly used for its digestive properties, particularly for the treatment of nausea and indigestion. Because of its ability to stimulate digestion and relieve nausea, ginger oil is frequently used as a treatment for morning sickness in pregnant women as well as motion sickness. Ginger oil can be inhaled or taken in diluted form because of these properties. Fennel oil, which has been used for centuries in many different cultures due to its carminative characteristics, is beneficial for relieving bloating and flatulence because it relaxes the muscles of the gastrointestinal tract and encourages the expulsion of gas. The use of these oils offers a comprehensive approach to digestive health, providing relief from discomfort while simultaneously supporting the natural digestive processes that occur within the body.

Perhaps one of the most common applications of oils is in the treatment of skin conditions and the care of the skin. For a very long time, essential oils derived from plants like lavender, tea tree, and chamomile have been utilized for the treatment of skin disorders such as acne, eczema, and infections. Little burns, cuts, and insect bites can all be effectively treated with lavender oil because of its calming and healing powers, which have earned it a well-deserved reputation. Because of its anti-inflammatory and antiseptic properties, it is frequently used as a treatment for acne, where it helps minimize the appearance of redness and swelling as well as the likelihood of infection. Also recognized for its antibacterial and antifungal effects, tea tree oil is another potent oil that has been used for centuries. Acne, athlete's foot, fungal infections, and dandruff are just some of the conditions that have been successfully treated with this substance. Studies conducted in clinical settings have proven that tea tree oil is beneficial in reducing acne lesions. This is attributed to the oil's capacity to eliminate germs that cause acne and to reduce inflammation. It is common practice to apply chamomile oil, which is well-known for its relaxing characteristics, to soothe skin that has been irritated, particularly in cases of eczema and dermatitis. Those who suffer from chronic skin diseases can get relief from their symptoms by using this product since its anti-inflammatory components assist in reducing skin redness, swelling, and itching. These oils provide a natural and gentle alternative to harsh chemical treatments, thereby promoting the health of the skin while also addressing a wide variety of skin problems.

It has been demonstrated that oils are useful in the management of pain, particularly in the relief of pain in the joints and muscles. Essential oils, like lavender, rosemary, and eucalyptus, have been found to be effective in treating a variety of ailments, including arthritis, muscular strains, and general aches and pains through their use. Because of its calming and anti-inflammatory characteristics, lavender oil is frequently utilized in massage therapy for the purpose of reducing tension and soothing muscles that are experiencing discomfort. In addition to its analgesic and anti-inflammatory properties, rosemary oil is a well-liked treatment for a variety of painful conditions, including arthritis, muscular stiffness, and joint pain. For the purpose of reducing inflammation and promoting circulation, it is frequently administered topically in conjunction with additional carrier oils. Due to the fact that it has qualities that are both cooling and anti-inflammatory, eucalyptus oil is commonly utilized in the treatment of joint pain and muscular soreness. In order to alleviate pain and speed up the healing process, it works by boosting the amount of blood that flows to the affected areas. The use of these oils in massage or as part of topical therapies offers a natural and effective method of pain management that does not require the use of artificial painkillers or anti-inflammatory medicines.

Additionally, oils have been shown to be incredibly beneficial in treating a variety of common ailments, including headaches and migraines. Since peppermint oil contains menthol, it is frequently used to alleviate headaches caused by tension, including migraines and tension headaches. Peppermint oil has a cooling impact that helps to relax tense muscles and promote circulation, which ultimately results in a reduction in headache discomfort. This effect can be found when the oil is applied topically to the temples or inhaled. The effectiveness of peppermint oil in lowering the severity of headaches has been demonstrated by studies to be comparable to that of acetaminophen. Moreover, lavender oil is frequently utilized for the purpose of alleviating headaches, particularly those that are brought on by tension or stress. Its relaxing and sedative effects assist in diminishing the intensity of headaches and induce relaxation, which is why it is a popular choice in aromatherapy for the treatment of headaches. Eucalyptus oil is useful in reducing sinus pressure and facilitating easier breathing, both of which can ease headache symptoms. This is especially true in situations where migraines are caused by sinus congestion or respiratory difficulties. These oils provide relief from pain while also addressing underlying causes such as tension or congestion, making them a natural alternative to non-prescription headache drugs that are available over the counter.

It has also been used to cure common disorders such as stress, anxiety, and depression. Another area where oils have been utilized to treat common ailments is emotional and mental health. Aromatherapy, which involves altering one's state of mind and feelings through the application of essential oils, has been an integral part of holistic healing methods for a very long time. It is common practice to use lavender oil, which is recognized for its calming effects, in order to alleviate feelings of stress and worry. Several studies have demonstrated that inhaling lavender oil can reduce levels of the stress hormone cortisol and induce relaxation, making it an effective treatment for mild to moderate anxiety. Bergamot oil, which is another essential oil that is often used in aromatherapy, is well-known for the elevating and mood-related properties that it possesses. In order to alleviate the symptoms of anxiety and depression, it is frequently utilized to foster a sense of tranquility and well-being in the individual. For the purpose of fostering mental clarity and emotional equilibrium, frankincense oil, which is highly regarded for its contemplative and grounding characteristics, is commonly utilized in spiritual practices and meditation programs. The use of these oils in aromatherapy or topical applications provides a natural and comprehensive approach to the management of stress and emotional well-being. This method offers an alternative to the use of pharmacological treatments for anxiety and depression.

In addition, oils have demonstrated considerable benefits when used in the treatment of sleep disorders. Sleep disorders, such as insomnia and poor sleep quality, are widespread conditions that affect millions of people all over the world. Essential oils like lavender, chamomile, and sandalwood have been used for a very long time to accomplish the goals of promoting restful sleep and improving the quality of sleep. The calming qualities of lavender oil, in particular, as well as its capacity to improve sleep, have been the subject of a significant amount of research. Inhaling lavender oil prior to going to bed has been demonstrated to improve the quality of sleep, lengthen the amount of time spent sleeping, and lessen the frequency and severity of symptoms associated with insomnia. Because of its calming and soothing effects, chamomile oil is frequently used to promote relaxation and reduce anxiety. As a result, it is a useful cure for sleep disturbances for those who suffer from these conditions. One of the most common uses of sandalwood oil in aromatherapy is to encourage deep sleep and to assist meditation practices. Sandalwood oil is known for its anchoring and meditative effects. In addition to increasing overall well-being and supporting the body's natural sleep-wake cycle, these oils provide a natural and efficient method of enhancing the quality of sleep without the need for prescription sleep aids.

Additionally, oils have been traditionally utilized to treat a variety of diseases, including those that affect women's health. In order to ease symptoms of premenstrual syndrome (PMS), menstrual cramps, and menopause, essential oils such as clary sage, lavender, and geranium have recently gained widespread popularity. Clary sage oil, which is well-known for its ability to provide hormonal equilibrium, is frequently utilized for the purpose of alleviating menstrual cramps and regulating hormonal variations that occur during the menstrual cycle. The symptoms of menopause, such as hot flashes and mood swings, can also be alleviated with the help of this substance. As a result of its relaxing and anti-inflammatory effects, lavender oil is frequently utilized for the purpose of alleviating menstrual cramps and promoting relaxation during the menstrual cycle. There is a common practice of using geranium oil to reduce symptoms of premenstrual syndrome (PMS) and menopause. These symptoms include mood swings, irritability, and bloating. Geranium oil is known for its balancing effects on the endocrine system. The use of these oils offers a natural and holistic approach to the management of women's health conditions, providing relief from discomfort while also promoting hormonal balance.

In conclusion, the utilization of oils as a modality for the treatment of common diseases has a strong foundation in both conventional medical procedures and contemporary holistic healing modalities. Oils provide a natural and effective alternative to synthetic pharmaceuticals for a variety of health conditions, including but not limited to respiratory health, digestive issues, skin care, pain management, emotional well-being, and women's health. It is because of their adaptability and capacity to treat a wide variety of health problems that they are an invaluable instrument for the management of common disorders and the promotion of overall health and well-being. It is likely that the role of oils in natural medicine will expand as research continues to validate the therapeutic properties of oils. Oils offer a holistic and accessible approach to treating common ailments, which is becoming increasingly important in a world that is looking for natural and sustainable health solutions.

Immune Support

It is a time-honored technique that has its origins in holistic healing traditions from a wide range of cultures all over the world to make use of essential oils for the purpose of bolstering the immune system. It has been known for a long time that essential oils, which are concentrated extracts of plants, have the potential to strengthen the immune system, prevent sickness, and facilitate overall wellness. These essential oils are obtained from plants that are well-known for their therapeutic capabilities, which include the ability to fight germs, viruses, fungi, and inflammation. The use of essential oils as an alternative or complement to conventional therapy for the purpose of promoting immune health has become increasingly popular as the interest in natural therapies has grown. Many of the immune-boosting advantages of these oils have been validated by modern science as study has progressed. This confirms the function that these oils play in strengthening the body's defenses and assisting in the prevention of infections and disorders.

The immune system is a complex network of organs, cells, and proteins that protects the body from infections, invading pathogens, and hazardous substances. Its primary function is to defend the body against these threats. It is critical for one's general health and well-being to keep their immune system in good shape. The immune system can be compromised by a number of causes, including but not limited to stress, failure to get enough sleep, poor food, exposure to environmental pollutants, and chronic illnesses. Essential oils have the potential to strengthen and increase immune function when they are utilized in the appropriate manner. This can assist the body in better resisting these assaults. Essential oils have the potential to offer a holistic approach to immunological health because of their capacity to lower inflammation, bring about relaxation, and combat infections.

Their antibacterial qualities are one of the key ways in which essential oils provide assistance to the immune system. It has been shown that a great number of essential oils have powerful antibacterial, antiviral, and antifungal properties, which can assist in protecting the body from germs that carry toxic properties. When it comes to antibacterial characteristics, tea tree oil, for instance, is well-known for its potency. Infections caused by bacteria and fungi have been the target of its use for ages, making it an extremely useful instrument for both the prevention and treatment of illness. Tea tree oil is a fantastic choice for strengthening immunological health because numerous studies have demonstrated that it is capable of successfully killing bacteria, viruses, and fungi.

The antibacterial and anti-inflammatory effects of eucalyptus oil, which is derived from the chemical eucalyptol, attract a lot of people to use it. In addition to promoting overall immune function, it has been demonstrated to assist in the elimination of respiratory infections, as well as to reduce inflammation in the airways.

Additionally, oregano oil is a well-known essential oil that is recognized for its immune-enhancing effects. The antibacterial and antiviral properties of oregano oil are aided by the presence of substances such as carvacrol and thymol. Traditional medical practitioners have employed it as a treatment for a variety of inflammatory conditions, including lung infections, digestive problems, and other diseases. One of the most effective natural remedies for warding off colds, the flu, and other diseases is oregano oil, which, according to research, can assist in the fight against harmful bacteria and viruses. The fact that it can strengthen the immune system by increasing the number of white blood cells and decreasing the amount of oxidative stress further emphasizes the significance of this substance in establishing and maintaining overall immunological health.

There are benefits linked with lavender oil that strengthen the immune system, despite the fact that it is commonly associated with relaxation and stress alleviation. Stress that lasts for an extended period of time is known to impair the immune system, which in turn makes the body more susceptible to infections and disorders. Indirectly aiding immune function, the relaxing and sedative effects of lavender oil help reduce stress levels, which in turn helps. Lavender oil assists the body in recovering from illness and bolsters its natural defenses by facilitating relaxation and producing better sleep. The production of cortisol, the stress hormone, which, when raised for extended periods of time, can depress the immune system, has been demonstrated to be reduced by lavender oil, according to research from the United States. Further supporting the health of the immune system is the fact that the anti-inflammatory and antioxidant properties of lavender oil assist in reducing inflammation in the body.

It has been discovered that frankincense oil, which existed in ancient cultures and was revered for its spiritual and therapeutic characteristics, can also improve immunological function. In addition to having powerful anti-inflammatory and antibacterial properties, the chemicals that are found in frankincense can also assist the body in warding off infections and reducing inflammation in the immune system. For centuries, aromatherapy has made use of it to improve respiratory health, lessen inflammation, and fortify the immune response that the body possesses. The generation of white blood cells, which are essential for the fight against infections and disorders, has been found to be stimulated by frankincense oil, according to many studies. A helpful tool for maintaining overall health and well-being, frankincense oil is a valuable tool because of its capacity to support the immune response of the body, as well as its relaxing and grounding properties.

Lemon oil is abundant in antioxidants and vitamin C, both of which are necessary for a healthy immune system. Lemon oil is another essential oil that is frequently used for the purpose of providing support to the immune system. Toxins and pathogens can be removed from the body with the help of lemon oil, which is known for its capacity to detoxify the body, increase circulation, and support lymphatic drainage. Due to the fact that it possesses antibacterial and antiviral qualities, it is also suitable for the prevention of infections, particularly those that impact the respiratory system. Lemon oil can be used to purify the air, minimize exposure to hazardous microorganisms, and promote a healthy immune response. It can also be applied topically and inhaled at the same time. The uplifting and stimulating characteristics of lemon oil can also help increase mood and mental clarity, which can have a favorable impact on immunological health. Lemon oil is a great antioxidant.

Thyme oil is yet another potent essential oil that is well-known for the bolstering effects it has on the immune system. Traditional medicine has been using thyme oil for generations to cure infections and strengthen the immune system. Thyme oil is rich in thymol, a chemical that has powerful antibacterial effects. One of the most powerful treatments for respiratory infections, skin disorders, and digestive issues is thyme oil because of its ability to fight bacteria, viruses, and fungi. For the purpose of warding off illnesses and ensuring that one's immune system remains robust, research has demonstrated that thyme oil has the ability to promote the creation of immune cells, such as white blood cells and T-cells. One further thing that demonstrates its involvement in supporting overall immune function is the fact that it can lower inflammation and help promote respiratory health.

There are immune-supportive effects associated with peppermint oil, which is often used for its refreshing and cooling characteristics. Additionally, peppermint oil contains menthol, which is a chemical that is well-known for its antibacterial and antiviral properties. Symptoms of the respiratory system that are associated with colds and the flu, such as congestion, coughing, and sore throat, are frequently alleviated by utilizing this substance. A powerful treatment for respiratory infections, peppermint oil, is able to remove mucus and reduce inflammation in the respiratory system, making it an excellent herbal cure. Additionally, the stimulating characteristics of peppermint oil can help enhance energy levels and improve mental clarity, both of which can indirectly support immunological health by reducing stress and energy levels.

On the other hand, clove oil, which is well-known for its powerful antibacterial and antioxidant qualities, is another essential oil that is frequently used to enhance the immune system. Eugenol, which is found in clove oil, is a chemical that has powerful benefits against bacteria, viruses, and inflammation. The treatment of infections, the reduction of inflammation, and the enhancement of immunological function are all areas in which it has been traditionally utilized in the medical field. Several studies have demonstrated that clove oil is capable of warding off pathogenic bacteria and viruses, making it an extremely useful instrument for both the prevention and treatment of diseases. The antioxidant qualities of clove oil also help reduce oxidative stress and inflammation in the body, which further supports the health of the immune system.

Essential oils have the ability to bolster immune function by aiding detoxification, in addition to their antibacterial and anti-inflammatory properties. Detoxification of the body and elimination of dangerous compounds that can impair the immune system are performed by the skin, the lymphatic system, and the liver, which are all crucial organs. In addition to their capacity to assist liver and lymphatic function, essential oils such as juniper berries, grapefruit, and rosemary are well-known for their cleansing effects. For instance, juniper berry oil possesses diuretic effects, which assist in the elimination of toxins from the body and bolster the functioning of the kidneys. It is a powerful therapy for detoxifying the body and supporting general immunological health since grapefruit oil is high in antioxidants and helps support liver function. Grapefruit oil supports liver function. In addition to enhancing immunological function, rosemary oil is well-known for its capacity to stimulate lymphatic drainage, which assists in the elimination of waste products and toxins from the body.

Furthermore, essential oils have the ability to improve gastrointestinal health, which in turn can help the immune system. Due to the fact that it is home to a significant number of immune cells in the body, the functioning of the immune system is greatly dependent on the gut. A compromised digestive tract can result in a compromised immune system, which in turn can lead to an increased likelihood of contracting infections and illnesses. It has been demonstrated that essential oils derived from herbs such as peppermint, ginger, and oregano can improve digestive health by lowering inflammation levels in the stomach, encouraging the growth of good bacteria, and warding off malicious pathogens. For instance, peppermint oil is well-known for its capacity to alleviate symptoms of irritable bowel syndrome (IBS) and to encourage healthy digestion, both of which can indirectly have a positive impact on immunological function. The anti-inflammatory characteristics of ginger oil can help reduce inflammation in the gut, which is one of the reasons why ginger oil is often used to treat digestive concerns such as nausea, indigestion, and bloating. By virtue of its potent antibacterial and antiviral properties, oregano oil has the potential to assist in the elimination of unwanted bacteria in the digestive tract, thereby fostering a balanced and healthy flora in the gut and bolstering the immune system.

Aromatherapy is another powerful method for bolstering the immune system, and it involves inhaling essential oils. These molecules move to the limbic system and the olfactory system in the brain when essential oils are inhaled. The limbic system is responsible for regulating emotions, stress levels, and immunological function, and it is directly affected by essential oils. Essential oils such as lavender, frankincense, and bergamot are frequently utilized in aromatherapy for the purpose of alleviating stress and anxiety, all of which have the potential to impair the immune system over periods of time. These oils have the potential to help boost the immune system and promote general health by lowering the body's stress response and inducing relaxation. As an additional means of bolstering immune function, the antibacterial qualities of particular essential oils can assist in the purification of the air and the reduction of exposure to hazardous pathogens.

Enhancing the health of the immune system can also be accomplished through the topical application of essential oils. Essential oils have the potential to make a direct impact on the immune system when they are absorbed into the bloodstream after being applied to the skin. In order to combat infections and bring down inflammation, it is usual practice to use oils such as tea tree, eucalyptus, and oregano on the skin. In order to improve lung health, enhance circulation, and support overall immunological function, these essential oils can be applied to the chest, back, or soles of the feet after being diluted in carrier oil. Massage treatment can also be used to enhance lymphatic drainage, reduce inflammation, and promote detoxification, all of which contribute to further boosting immunological health. Certain essential oils can be used in massage therapy.

For the purpose of bolstering the immune system and promoting overall health and well-being, essential oils provide a method that is both natural and efficient. When it comes to preventing and treating infections, lowering inflammation, and promoting detoxification, they are extremely useful tools due to their antibacterial, anti-inflammatory, and detoxifying qualities. Essential oils can help boost the body's defenses and improve immunological function by promoting healthier respiratory and digestive functions, as well as reducing stress levels. Essential oils are anticipated to play an increasingly vital role in promoting immune health and overall wellness as the interest in alternative therapies continues to develop among people. The use of essential oils, on the other hand, must be done so in a manner that is both safe and suitable. Certain oils have the potential to be toxic or to provoke allergic reactions if they are utilized in excessive quantities or without the right dilution. It is possible to ensure the safe and successful use of essential oils for immune support by consulting with a healthcare practitioner or an aromatherapist who is certified.

Skin and Hair Care

Over the course of several centuries, skin and hair care have been fundamental components of beauty and health routines in a variety of different cultures. Essential oils and carrier oils have been appreciated for their medicinal capabilities for a very long time. They have also been utilized to promote good skin and hair for a very long time. These natural oils, which are obtained from plants, seeds, nuts, and flowers, include a wide range of vitamins, antioxidants, and nutrients that have the potential to nourish, renew, and protect the skin and hair. These oils are appealing because of their adaptability; they can be used to treat a wide variety of skin and hair disorders, ranging from dryness to acne to hair loss. This versatility is what makes these oils so appealing. The current beauty industry has embraced the use of oils in skincare and haircare products as a result of the growing number of individuals who are looking for natural alternatives to products that are synthetic and include a lot of chemicals. As a consequence of this, oils have evolved as potent and effective tools for the purpose of preserving the vitality and health of both my hair and my skin.

The moisturizing effect of oils is one of the most well-known applications of oils in skin care. When it comes to regulating moisture levels and delivering hydration to the skin, oils are among the best options. Because they provide a barrier that prevents water loss from the skin, oils like jojoba, argan, and coconut are commonly used as moisturizers. This is because these oils build a protective barrier on the skin. Because it is so similar to the sebum that is naturally produced by the skin, jojoba oil, for instance, is particularly useful for hydrating the skin without causing the pores to become clogged. Because of its high concentration of vital fatty acids and vitamin E, argan oil, which is frequently referred to as "liquid gold," is able to supply the skin with intense hydration and rebuild the skin's moisture barrier. Coconut oil, which is well-known for its ability to deeply moisturize the skin, has been utilized for a long time in tropical regions as a multifunctional oil for the care of both the skin and the hair. When these oils are applied to the skin, they not only hydrate the skin but also offer a protective barrier that guards the skin against environmental aggressors such as pollution, ultraviolet radiation, and harsh weather conditions.

While essential oils and carrier oils are commonly used for their moisturizing characteristics, they are also widely used for their anti-aging properties. As people become older, their skin loses its elasticity, firmness, and hydration, which results in the appearance of wrinkles, fine lines, and sagging skin. The capacity of certain oils, such as rosehip, frankincense, and pomegranate, to minimize the appearance of signs of aging has earned them a lot of praise. Rosehip oil, which is abundant in vitamins A and C, is known to stimulate the formation of collagen, which is a vital component in the process of preserving the suppleness and firmness of the skin. Additionally, this oil is loaded with antioxidants, which are known to counteract free radicals, which are the agents that are responsible for the breakdown of collagen and elastin. Because of the revitalizing properties that it has on the skin, frankincense oil has been utilized for this purpose by ancient civilizations for ages. It helps to reduce the look of wrinkles and age spots while also helping to tone and lift skin that has become drooping. With its high concentration of antioxidants and polyphenols, pomegranate oil helps to shield the skin from the damaging effects of oxidative stress and encourages the regeneration of skin cells. The constant application of these oils has the potential to assist in the smoothing of the skin, the reduction of the appearance of fine lines and wrinkles, and the promotion of a complexion that is more youthful and radiant.

Another area in which essential oils have been shown to be useful is acne, which is a prevalent skin condition that affects people of all ages. Acne is frequently brought on by an overabundance of sebum production, pores that are clogged, and the growth of bacteria on the skin as a result of its antibacterial, anti-inflammatory, and antiseptic characteristics, tea tree oil is widely considered to be one of the most effective essential oils for treating acne. Tea tree oil, when applied to the skin, helps destroy germs that cause acne, reduce inflammation, and dry up pimples without causing the skin to become overly dry. Additionally, lavender oil, which is an essential oil that possesses anti-inflammatory and antibacterial qualities, has the ability to calm skin that has been irritated and lessen the redness that is associated with acne. Additionally, despite the fact that it is an oil, jojoba oil has the ability to help control the natural oil production of the skin, making it an excellent option for people who have oily skin or skin that is very prone to acne. The production of sebum is brought into balance by these oils, which helps avoid clogged pores and breakouts, resulting in skin that is both clearer and healthier.

There are a number of other skin problems that can be effectively treated with oils, including psoriasis and eczema. It can be especially challenging to treat eczema, which is a persistent skin ailment that is characterized by dryness, itching, and inflammation of the skin. Evening primrose oil and borage oil are two examples of carrier oils that have a high concentration of gamma-linolenic acid (GLA), an important fatty acid that has been shown to reduce inflammation and increase the skin's ability to retain moisture. When these oils are applied to the affected regions, they assist in relieving itching, alleviating inflammation, and promoting healing. Individuals who suffer from eczema may also find relief from the condition through the use of essential oils like chamomile and lavender, which have the ability to calm the skin and reduce inflammation. In addition, the use of oils such as neem and tea tree can be beneficial for the treatment of psoriasis, which is another chronic skin disorder that results in the rapid accumulation of skin cells, which in turn produces scaling and irritation. Psoriasis is characterized by scaling and itching, both of which can be alleviated by using neem oil, which was discovered to have antifungal and anti-inflammatory qualities. As a result of its antibacterial characteristics, tea tree oil can be of assistance in preventing infections in areas of skin that have been broken. The combination of these oils has the potential to effectively treat the symptoms of certain persistent skin disorders and to improve the general health of the skin.

As with skin care, there has been an increase in interest in the utilization of oils for hair care as well. The nourishing, moisturizing, and protecting characteristics of oils are beneficial to the hair, just as they are to the skin when it comes to hair care. The promotion of hair growth and the reduction of hair loss are two of the most prominent applications of oils in the field of hair care. In order to treat hair thinning and hair loss, castor oil, which is abundant in ricinoleic acid and omega-6 fatty acids, is frequently utilized as a therapeutic component. The application of castor oil to the scalp in the form of a massage helps to stimulate blood circulation, which in turn promotes hair growth and strengthens the hair follicles. Additionally, rosemary oil is an essential oil that has been demonstrated to stimulate hair follicles and improve circulation to the scalp, both of which are known to be beneficial to hair development. According to a number of studies, rosemary oil may be just as efficient as minoxidil, which is a common prescription used to cure hair loss; however, rosemary oil does not have any negative side effects.

Furthermore, oils have the potential to enhance the overall health and appearance of the hair, in addition to their ability to stimulate hair growth. For example, coconut oil is frequently utilized as a means of providing the hair with a thorough conditioner. Because of its small molecular structure, it is able to permeate the hair shaft, making it possible to provide profound hydration and reduce the loss of protein. Coconut oil is very good for people who have dry hair, hair that has been damaged by chemicals, or hair that has been treated with chemicals. Due to the high levels of vital fatty acids and vitamin E that it contains, argan oil is frequently utilized for the purpose of imparting shine and smoothness to the hair. There is a reduction in frizz, protection against heat damage caused by styling equipment, and nourishment of the hair, which results in the hair being softer, more lustrous, and easier to manage.

Fundamental oils have the potential to play a significant part in the process of developing and sustaining a healthy scalp, which is another fundamental component of hair care. A healthy scalp is necessary for the growth of hair as well as the overall health of the hair. Tea tree oil and peppermint oil are two examples of oils that are well-known for their capacity to cleanse and detoxify the scalp. A number of scalp problems, including dandruff and seborrheic dermatitis, can be treated with tea tree oil due to its antibacterial and antifungal qualities. These properties allow tea tree oil to eliminate the fungus that is responsible for these conditions. Due to the fact that it has a cooling and calming effect, peppermint oil can assist in reducing inflammation and irritation of the scalp while simultaneously increasing circulation. Utilizing these oils on a consistent basis can assist in the maintenance of a healthy scalp, the prevention of dandruff, and the promotion of stronger, healthier hair.

In addition to these popular uses, oils have a wide range of other applications in the care of both the skin and the hair. For instance, oils derived from calendula and chamomile are widely utilized in formulations that are supposed to be relaxing and therapeutic for skin that is either sensitive or inflamed. It is common practice to apply calendula oil to the treatment of minor wounds such as cuts, scrapes, and burns, as well as skin disorders such as dermatitis and eczema. Calendula oil is known for its therapeutic and anti-inflammatory effects. It is common practice to incorporate chamomile oil into skincare products developed for sensitive skin because of its ability to reduce redness and irritation. Chamomile oil is known for its relaxing and anti-inflammatory properties.

Similarly, oils such as grapeseed and almonds are frequently utilized in the creation of hair care products since they offer a lightweight hydration that does not cause the hair to get weighed down. Because it is abundant in vitamins A and E, almond oil is beneficial for nourishing the scalp and hair, as well as increasing the suppleness and gloss of the hair. Because of the high concentration of linoleic acid that it contains, grapeseed oil is an ideal option for people who have oily hair because it hydrates the hair without leaving it greasy or weighed down.

It is one of the reasons that oils have become such an important component of beauty routines all around the world that they are so versatile in terms of their application to both skincare and hair care. It doesn't matter if you use oils as moisturizers, anti-aging treatments, acne solutions, or hair growth stimulants; oils provide a natural and efficient way to enhance beauty and support overall skin and hair health. Because an increasing number of people are looking for natural alternatives to conventional beauty products, it is probable that oils will continue to play a big role in the skincare and haircare routines of individuals.

On the other hand, it is essential to make appropriate use of oils in order to prevent any potential unwanted reactions or side effects. Because of the high concentration of certain oils, particularly essential oils, it is necessary to dilute them with a carrier oil before applying them to the skin or hair. Additionally, persons who have sensitive skin or specific skin conditions should perform a patch test prior to using a new oil in order to verify that they do not develop an adverse reaction to the oil. For the purpose of ensuring the safe and effective utilization of oils in skincare and haircare regimens, it is advisable to seek the advice of a professional aromatherapist or a cosmetic dermatologist.

In addition to its widespread application in moisturizing, anti-aging, and the treatment of skin disorders, oils also provide substantial benefits in the protection of skin and hair from the damaging effects of adverse environmental conditions. Many oils include natural antioxidants, which defend the skin and hair against damage caused by pollution, ultraviolet rays, and other environmental factors. These antioxidants help neutralize free radicals and protect the skin and hair from harm. Pomegranate seed oil, for example, contains a high concentration of antioxidants like polyphenols and vitamin C, both of which assist in protecting the skin from the damaging effects of oxidative stress and environmental contaminants. In a similar vein, avocado oil, which is laden with antioxidants such as vitamin E and carotenoids, offers significant protection against sun damage. It does this by assisting in the absorption of ultraviolet radiation and avoiding damage caused by free radicals, which can potentially lead to premature aging.

When it comes to protecting the skin and hair from the elements, the capacity of oils to create a natural barrier is especially important in areas that experience extreme weather conditions. In cold and dry settings, where the skin has a tendency to lose moisture fast, oils like olive oil and shea butter can work as emollients, preventing chapping, cracking, and irritation by locking in moisture and keeping the skin from drying out. Shea butter, which is abundant in vitamins A and E as well as fatty acids, has been utilized for a very long time in African cultures as a means of shielding the skin from the intense heat of the desert environment. Olive oil is another traditional medicine that has been used for centuries because of its ability to moisturize and preserve the skin. In addition to hydrating the skin, it also forms a barrier that helps protect the skin from the elements, such as wind and cold.

Coconut oil and tamanu oil are two examples of oils that can be used to protect the skin and hair from excessive moisture loss and environmental contaminants. These oils are particularly useful in tropical areas, which are characterized by increased exposure to the sun and humidity. Because of its high concentration of medium-chain fatty acids, coconut oil is a well-liked option for tropical hair care because it is particularly excellent in protecting the hair from the effects of humidity and reducing frizz. Because of its capacity to treat and protect the skin from sunburns, wounds, and irritations, tamarind oil, which is indigenous to Southeast Asia, has gained a lot of popularity. In the past, people from the Pacific Islands have used it to protect and nourish their skin after being exposed to the sun and seawater for an extended period of time.

Oils are also an important component in the treatment of hyperpigmentation and uneven skin tone, both of which are conditions that are experienced by a large number of people all over the world. A number of factors, including sun exposure, hormone shifts, acne scars, and inflammation, can all contribute to hyperpigmentation. It is well known that certain oils, such as rosehip and carrot seed, have the capacity to brighten the skin and level out the tone of the skin. Through its ability to stimulate the turnover of skin cells and the creation of collagen, rosehip oil, which is abundant in retinoids and vitamin C, helps to lessen the visibility of scars and dark spots on the skin. Through the process of boosting the regeneration of skin cells, carrot seed oil, which is rich in beta-carotene and vitamin A, helps to reduce hyperpigmentation and enhance the overall tone of the skin.

The use of style tools, chemical treatments, and environmental stress can all cause damage to the hair, which can be mitigated by incorporating oils into your shampoo and conditioner routines. Grapeseed oil and argan oil are two examples of oils that are widely used as heat protectants. These oils are applied to the hair in order to shield it from the damage that is caused by blow dryers, curling irons, and flat irons. Because of its high smoke point, grapeseed oil is able to form a protective barrier around the hair shaft, thus avoiding the loss of moisture and damage that might occur as a result of heat styling. Because of the high concentration of essential fatty acids and antioxidants that it contains, argan oil not only shields the hair from the damaging effects of heat but also repairs and strengthens damaged strands, thereby restoring luster and softness.

The use of oils can also be beneficial to hair color treatments since oils help to preserve the luster and health of hair that has been colored. In addition to making the hair more prone to breakage, dryness, and dullness, chemical dyes, and bleaches can also cause the hair to become weaker. Jojoba and olive oils are two examples of oils that can be used to restore moisture to color-treated hair and protect it from fading. These oils can also help nourish and maintain color-treated hair. Jojoba oil, which is very similar to the natural oils that are found on the scalp, helps to maintain a healthy balance of moisture on the scalp and safeguards against dryness, which can result in the loss of color. Because of its conditioning capabilities, olive oil helps strengthen and soften hair that has been chemically treated, which in turn makes the hair less likely to split into pieces.

Individuals who have curly or textured hair can benefit from using oils because they offer a natural method to improve the definition of their curls, add shine, and minimize frizz. Because the natural oils that are produced by the scalp have a more difficult time going down the hair shaft, curly hair has a tendency to be drier and more prone to frizz than straight hair. The moisture and nutrients that are necessary for the maintenance of healthy curls can be acquired through the use of oils such as coconut and castor oil. Because it is able to penetrate the hair shaft, coconut oil is able to provide intense moisture and reduce the loss of protein, both of which are vital for the maintenance of curls that are strong and defined. The thick nature of castor oil helps to seal in moisture and form a protective barrier that keeps curls hydrated and free of frizz. Castor oil is known for its capacity to produce a barrier.

In addition to addressing basic cosmetic concerns, oils are also utilized in luxury and spa treatments. These treatments make use of oils because of their aromatic and therapeutic capabilities, which are prized for their ability to promote relaxation and improve general well-being. Because of the calming and soothing effects that essential oils like lavender, chamomile, and sandalwood have on the mind and body, they are frequently utilized in massage therapy and beauty treatments. When it comes to facials and body treatments at spas, lavender oil is frequently utilized because of its calming and relaxing effects. This helps to calm the skin and encourage relaxation. Because of its anti-inflammatory characteristics, chamomile oil is frequently included in treatments for skin that is sensitive or irritated. This helps to soothe and calm redness on the skin. Sandalwood oil, which is highly regarded for its calming and contemplative properties, is frequently utilized in aromatherapy massages for the purpose of both alleviating tension and fostering a sense of inner peace.

Oils have been used for centuries in traditional practices for both haircare and skincare, but contemporary science has begun to prove their effectiveness through research and clinical investigations. Oils have been used for both haircare and skincare procedures. Extensive research has demonstrated that several oils possess powerful antibacterial, antifungal, and anti-inflammatory qualities. These properties enable these oils to effectively treat a wide variety of skin and hair disorders. The antibacterial qualities of tea tree oil, for instance, have been the subject of much research, and for this reason, it is frequently employed in the treatment of acne, dandruff, and fungal infections. Similarly, research has shown that argan oil can improve the flexibility of the skin and reduce the indications of aging. Coconut oil, on the other hand, has been demonstrated to increase the condition of the hair and reduce the amount of protein that is lost from the hair.

A number of changes in formulations have been brought about as a result of the increasing use of oils in contemporary skincare and haircare products. These developments involve the combination of oils with other natural components in order to produce beauty treatments that are both powerful and effective. Facial oils, for instance, frequently bring together a number of different oils, such as rosehip, jojoba, and argan, in order to produce a synergistic mixture that simultaneously tackles a number of different skin conditions. Additionally, hair serums typically include a combination of oils such as coconut, argan, and grapeseed in order to offer a comprehensive treatment that addresses hydration, frizz control, and heat protection for the hair.

It is essential to keep in mind that not all oils are appropriate for every type of skin or hair, despite the fact that oils offer a considerable number of advantages. Additionally, individuals who have oily or acne-prone skin may find that certain oils, particularly heavier oils such as coconut and olive, are too occlusive for their skin, which can result in clogged pores and outbreaks. Because they do not leave behind a greasy residue, lighter oils like grapeseed and jojoba are better suitable for oily or combination skin types. These oils moisturize the skin without leaving behind a greasy residue. Similarly, several essential oils have the potential to irritate the skin or trigger allergic reactions, particularly in people who have skin that is exceptionally sensitive. It is always suggested to perform a patch test before attempting to use a new oil in order to guarantee that it does not create an unfavorable reaction.

To summarize, the utilization of oils in the treatment of skin and hair is a time-honored practice that is continuously gaining favor as a result of the significant number of advantages that oils provide. The use of oils offers a natural and efficient solution for a wide variety of beauty difficulties, including the treatment of acne and the promotion of hair development, as well as the functions of moisturizing and anti-aging. Because of the abundance of vitamins, antioxidants, and vital fatty acids that they contain, they are extremely effective agents for nourishing, protecting, and regenerating the skin and hair from the inside out. Oils have the potential to revolutionize beauty routines and improve the general health of the skin and hair, regardless of whether they are used on their own or in conjunction with other natural substances. Oils will continue to be an essential component of both conventional and contemporary methods of haircare and skincare practice since they provide a holistic approach to beauty and well-being. This is because the demand for natural beauty products is expected to continue to grow.

CHAPTER IV

Oils for Mental and Emotional Well-being

Stress and Anxiety Reduction

In today's fast-paced and demanding environment, stress and anxiety have become widespread problems that affect people everywhere. Because of the growing number of people who are concerned about their mental health, more and more people are looking for natural and holistic treatments to alleviate the stresses of contemporary life. Additionally, the utilization of essential oils and oils derived from plants has emerged as a potent and natural alternative among the numerous methods that are available for the alleviation of stress and anxiety. From ancient Egypt, India, and China, where oils were included in everyday rituals, religious rites, and healing procedures, the practice of utilizing oils for stress management extends back thousands of years. This practice has been handed down from generation to generation. Due to the fact that the therapeutic effects of oils are now recognized and proven by scientific studies, they have become a popular choice among persons who are looking for a holistic approach to the management of anxiety and stress in their lives.

Aromatherapy, which involves the inhalation of essential oils to stimulate the olfactory system, is one of the most significant ways that oils can alleviate stress. Aromatherapy is commonly used in the United States. When essential oils are inhaled, the chemicals in them come into contact with receptors in the nose. These receptors are connected to the limbic system, which is the region of the brain that is responsible for controlling emotions, behavior, and cognitive processes. Because of this direct interaction, essential oils are able to exert an influence on the emotional center of the brain, which results in effects that are calming and relaxing. Lavender, chamomile, and bergamot oils are particularly well-known for their capacity to alleviate anxiety, quiet the nervous system, and induce a sensation of relaxation. Also noted for their ability to promote relaxation. In particular, lavender has been the subject of a significant amount of research for its ability to alleviate anxiety. It has been demonstrated via research that lavender oil has the ability to lower levels of cortisol, which is the hormone that is responsible for stress and provides a relaxing impact on the neurological system. This can help reduce anxiety and enhance mood.

In addition to its long-standing association with relaxation and the ability to soothe the mind, chamomile oil has also been demonstrated to possess anti-anxiety qualities. Apigenin is a naturally occurring chemical that binds to GABA receptors in the brain, providing calming effects that are comparable to those of prescribed anti-anxiety drugs. Chamomile's ability to alleviate anxiety can be ascribed to the high concentration of apigenin that it contains. When it comes to aromatherapy, chamomile oil is frequently utilized to alleviate the symptoms of anxiety, provide assistance with insomnia, and encourage relaxation before going to bed. Chamomile is an excellent option for people who suffer from nervous tension and chronic stress because of its beneficial characteristics, which include calming and relaxing effects.

Another oil that possesses potent anti-anxiety effects is bergamot, which is a citrus oil that has a fragrance that is both invigorating and fresh. The levels of the stress hormone cortisol can be lowered, and a sensation of calm can be induced by bergamot oil, according to studies. Bergamot oil can greatly reduce stress and anxiety. Along with helping to enhance mood and lessen feelings of despair, which are frequently connected with chronic stress and worry, its pleasant aroma also helps to boost mood. Bergamot oil is frequently utilized in diffusers, massage blends, and bath products with the purpose of producing an environment that is both calming and aids in alleviating tension. Because it has the power to bring about a state of equilibrium in mood and to alleviate emotional tension, it is a wonderful option for people who are coping with stress, anxiety, and mood swings.

Furthermore, rose oil is another essential oil that is well-known for its ability to alleviate tension. Researchers have discovered that the sweet and floral aroma of rose oil can reduce levels of the stress hormone cortisol and provide a relaxing impact on the neurological system. Research has demonstrated that rose oil has the potential to considerably alleviate symptoms of anxiety and depression, particularly in people who are under a significant amount of stress on a regular basis. It is common practice to incorporate rose oil into aromatherapy, bath products, and massage oils in order to facilitate relaxation and alleviate emotional strain. Its calming aroma not only helps to settle the mind but also delivers a sense of emotional comfort, which is why it is such a popular choice for people who are struggling with sorrow, despair, or emotional upheaval.

Essential oil mixes, in addition to the individual oils listed above, are frequently utilized for the purpose of alleviating stress and anxiety conditions. When it comes to fostering relaxation and establishing an atmosphere that is conducive to relaxation, blends that include essential oils such as lavender, chamomile, sandalwood, and frankincense are particularly useful. In religious and spiritual activities, frankincense oil has been treasured for a long time because of its grounding effect, which helps relieve tension and promotes a sense of inner calm or tranquility. It is possible for frankincense to increase the overall therapeutic advantages and produce a more profound sense of relaxation when it is taken in conjunction with other oils that contain relaxing properties.

In addition to the inhalation of oils conducted through aromatherapy, the application of oils to the skin can also be beneficial in reducing feelings of stress and anxiety. Essential oils, when applied to the skin, are absorbed into the bloodstream and come into contact with the various systems of the body, which results in the production of soothing symptoms. One of the most effective ways to alleviate stress and anxiety is through the practice of massage therapy, which combines the physical relaxing of muscle tension with the therapeutic effects of oils. A massage is a form of massage that has the ability to stimulate circulation, relax muscles, and promote the production of endorphins, which are the natural "feel-good" hormones present in the body. When massage is paired with calming oils such as lavender or chamomile, the effects of massage are amplified, resulting in a more profound state of relaxation and a reduction in stress.

In addition to aromatherapy and massage, the benefits of oils for reducing stress and anxiety are not restricted to these two practices. When it comes to promoting mental well-being, there are numerous oils that may be included in everyday routines in a variety of different ways. At the conclusion of a hard day, for instance, oils can be added to bath water to produce an experience that is both calming and relaxing for the individual. Taking a bath in warm water that has been infused with essential oils is an effective way to relax the mind, relieve tension in the muscles, and get the body ready for bed. It is usual practice to incorporate essential oils such as lavender, sandalwood, and eucalyptus into bath mixtures in order to provide a soothing environment and encourage relaxation.

It is also possible to use diffusers to create a calm atmosphere in the house or at the place of employment by using essential oils. Inhaling essential oils such as bergamot, cedarwood, or clary sage through a diffuser can be an effective method for alleviating stress and establishing a tranquil environment that fosters concentration and emotional equilibrium. This is especially helpful for people who are experiencing stress as a result of their work or who need to establish a calm environment in which they can meditate and relax.

Certain oils, in addition to their relaxing effects, also possess adaptogenic features, which means that they assist the body in adjusting to higher levels of stress and regaining its equilibrium. It is well recognized that certain oils, such as clary sage, vetiver, and ylang-ylang, have the capacity to assist the body's stress response and to boost emotional resilience. Clary sage, for example, has been demonstrated to lower cortisol levels and induce feelings of relaxation. As a result, it is an ideal choice for alleviating stress-related symptoms such as headaches and tension. As a result of its earthy and grounding aroma, vetiver is frequently utilized for the purpose of calming the mind and alleviating the symptoms of anxiety. Its rich, woodsy aroma contributes to the creation of a sense of stability and grounding, which can be especially good for people who are feeling overwhelmed or scattered as a result of stress.

As a result of its sweet and floral aroma, ylang-ylang is frequently utilized for the purpose of achieving emotional equilibrium and alleviating sensations of stress and worry. According to research, ylang-ylang has the ability to reduce blood pressure and generate a sense of peace. As a result, it is especially beneficial for people who experience physical symptoms of stress, such as a quick heartbeat or high blood pressure. In the context of emotional healing methods, ylang-ylang is frequently utilized to facilitate the discharge of negative emotions such as anger, irritation, and irritability.

The potential of oils to promote peaceful sleep is yet another manner in which they contribute to the reduction of stress and anxiety. It is common for insufficient sleep to be both a symptom and a source of stress and worry, thereby establishing a vicious cycle that can be challenging to stop. It is well known that certain oils, such as lavender, chamomile, and sandalwood, have calming effects, which serve to promote peaceful sleep and prevent the occurrence of insomnia. The ability of lavender oil, in particular, to improve the quality of sleep has been the subject of a significant amount of research. The inhalation of lavender oil prior to going to bed has been shown to improve the quality of sleep overall, as well as the duration of sleep, and to reduce the number of awakenings that occur during the night. Those persons who suffer from anxiety-induced insomnia or sleeplessness as a result of stress will find this to be of great benefit.

There is also chamomile oil, which is another oil that helps with relaxation and sleep. Chamomile, which is well-known for its mild sedative properties, is beneficial for unwinding the nervous system and getting the body ready for sleep. Before going to bed, chamomile tea, which is frequently consumed as part of a bedtime ritual, can be improved by adding a few drops of chamomile oil to a diffuser or by applying it directly to the skin. Not only does the relaxing effects of chamomile increase the quality of sleep, but they also assist lessen the symptoms of anxiety and nervous tension.

Additionally, due to the grounding and contemplative properties that it possesses, sandalwood oil is an effective tool for aiding deep sleep. Because of its perfume, which is rich and woodsy, it helps to calm the mind and create an atmosphere that is pleasant, which makes it easier to fall asleep and stay asleep. Individuals who suffer from racing thoughts or worry that stops them from getting a good night's sleep might benefit greatly from the capacity of sandalwood to relax the mind and minimize mental chatter more than anybody else.

Since the beginning of this century, scientific research has started to support the use of essential oils for the relief of stress and anxiety, further solidifying the position that essential oils play in contemporary health practices. Essential oils have been demonstrated to dramatically alleviate the symptoms of anxiety and increase general well-being, according to research conducted in clinical settings in many countries. For instance, a study that was carried out on individuals who were scheduled to undergo surgical procedures discovered that inhaling lavender oil before surgery caused a reduction in anxiety and an improvement in mood. In a similar vein, a study conducted on people who suffered from generalized anxiety disorder discovered that bergamot oil effectively alleviated the symptoms of anxiety, as well as improved overall mood and mental well-being.

Essential oils, in addition to their psychological impacts, also have physical advantages that can help relieve the physical symptoms of stress. These benefits can be found using essential oils. Due to the fact that many essential oils possess anti-inflammatory and pain-relieving characteristics, they are beneficial in alleviating tension headaches, muscle discomfort, and other physical symptoms that are associated with stress. One example is peppermint oil, which is well-known for its capacity to alleviate tension headaches and reduce muscle tension. As a result, it is a favorite choice among people who feel physical symptoms of stress. A cooling sensation is produced by peppermint oil when it is applied topically. This sensation helps reduce pain and relax tight muscles, which in turn promotes overall relaxation and stress alleviation.

In a similar vein, oils such as eucalyptus and rosemary are well-known for their capacity to alleviate pain and reduce inflammation. Muscle discomfort, joint stiffness, and tension headaches are common conditions that can be alleviated with the usage of eucalyptus oil due to its beneficial effects of cooling and calming. As a result of its analgesic and anti-inflammatory properties, rosemary oil is a useful cure for stress-related physical discomfort since it facilitates the reduction of pain and the improvement of circulation.

The journey toward lowering stress and anxiety is ultimately a personal one and different people may have different reactions to the various oils and methods that are available. Experimenting with a variety of oils and mixtures can assist folks in determining which ones meet their needs the most effectively. The habit of keeping a journal to record one's emotional reactions and physical feelings while using essential oils can be an extremely beneficial one, as it assists individuals in better comprehending their own requirements and preferences. Individuals have the ability to make personalized blends that resonate with their own emotional and physical requirements because of the huge assortment of oils that are available to them.

This age-old practice appears to have a bright future ahead of it as more and more research is being conducted on the effectiveness of essential oils in reducing tension and anxiety. Individuals can uncover the secrets of nature's healing abilities by incorporating the usage of oils into their everyday lives. By doing so, they can harness the therapeutic advantages of oils to build a stronger sense of peace, tranquility, and emotional resilience. A sanctuary of peace is provided by the simplicity and beauty of essential oils, which serve as a reminder of the significance of self-care and emotional well-being in our day-to-day lives. This is especially important in a world that frequently appears to be chaotic and all-encompassing. When we embrace the power of oils, we are not just providing relief from stress and anxiety; we are also providing nourishment to the body, mind, and spirit, so building a more profound connection to both ourselves and the world that surrounds us. Individuals are able to rediscover their inner calm, establish emotional equilibrium, and survive in the face of the obstacles that life presents when they can discover the secrets that nature has to offer.

Mood Enhancement

Enhancing one's mood is an essential component of overall well-being, which encompasses emotional steadiness, mental clarity, and psychological wellness. In today's fast-paced culture, where there is an abundance of pressures, it is essential to discover approaches that are helpful in elevating mood and cultivating positive emotions in order to live a life that is meaningful. The utilization of essential oils and oils derived from plants is among the most compelling and natural methods for enhancing one's mood. For millennia, people from a wide variety of cultures have been making use of these oils for their therapeutic properties, particularly in the realm of mental health. Essential oils are being increasingly recognized as beneficial aids in mood enhancement, as evidenced by the growing body of research that investigates the psychological and physiological effects of essential oils.

The limbic system of the brain, which is responsible for the regulation of emotions and memories, is closely tied to the olfactory system, which is responsible for our sense of smell. Aromatic molecules derived from essential oils are delivered to the olfactory receptors through the nasal cavity when the essential oils are breathed in. The limbic system is then reached by these chemicals, which transmit impulses. Because of this direct method of touch, essential oils have the ability to change our feelings, reduce tension, and boost our mood simultaneously. Lavender, citrus oils, and ylang-ylang are some of the oils that are particularly well-known for their uplifting properties. In addition to its well-known beneficial effects on relaxation, lavender also possesses mood-enhancing properties that can assist in alleviating feelings of anxiety and hopelessness. For example, it has been established that the calming floral aroma of lavender can reduce the levels of stress hormones in the body, which in turn contributes to emotions of peace and overall prosperity.

Citrus essential oils, which include lemon, orange, and bergamot, are known to have fragrances that are both stimulating and reviving. As a result, these oils appear to be particularly effective in improving one's mood. Serotonin is a neurotransmitter that is related to emotions of happiness and well-being. These oils are known to increase serotonin levels for this reason. Research, for example, found that breathing lemon essential oil led to elevated levels of serotonin, which in turn resulted in a noticeable improvement in temperament. When it comes to persons who are experiencing stress and depression, bergamot oil has been associated with lowering levels of anxiety and increasing mood. Because of their energizing and zesty aroma, citrus oils are perfect for diffusing in homes and workplaces since they not only invigorate the senses but also produce an environment that is filled with happiness and excitement.

Other effective mood enhancers include ylang-ylang oil, which is extracted from the blossoms of the Cananga tree. Aromatherapy has been utilized to relieve anxiety and establish emotional equilibrium through the application of its sweet and floral fragrance. "Ylang-ylang" oil has been shown to have a relaxing impact, which helps ease feelings of tension and stress. Research suggests that it can drop blood pressure and heart rate, generating a calming effect. Ylang-ylang is a versatile oil that can be used to promote emotional well-being because, in addition to its relaxing characteristics, it is also noted for its ability to enhance mood. When combined with other oils that are known to be uplifting, such as bergamot and orange, it can provide a synergy that is quite effective in elevating one's mood.

Not only may essential oils be inhaled to improve one's mood, but they can also be applied topically, which is another strategy that has proven to be successful. Essential oils are absorbed into the bloodstream when they are applied to the skin, which enables their ability to exert their medicinal effects. It is possible to achieve a dual advantage of relaxation and mood enhancement by massaging oils such as sweet almond, jojoba, or coconut oil that have been combined with essential oils that strengthen the mood. In order to alleviate stress and foster a sense of peace and tranquility, for example, a soothing mixture of lavender and chamomile oils can be massaged into the temples and the neck.

There are certain essential oils that, in addition to their psychological impacts, can also support the physical components of maintaining a positive mood. It is well known that essential oils such as rosemary and peppermint can stimulate the senses and promote mental clarity. In addition to enhancing cognitive performance, rosemary oil has been demonstrated to boost memory and promote alertness. Its aroma is described as being fresh and herbal. When it comes to activities that demand focus and concentration, rosemary oil is a good choice because it can be used to create an environment that is stimulating and stimulates creativity and mental agility.

By fostering feelings of alertness and vitality, peppermint oil, which is well-known for its aroma that is both invigorating and energizing, can also improve one's mood. One of the best ways to battle symptoms of exhaustion or mental sluggishness is to use peppermint oil, which has a cooling sensation that helps stimulate the mind. People who want to improve their mood and energy levels throughout the day may find that peppermint oil, whether it is used topically, diffused, or inhaled, is a fantastic tool to utilize.

The use of essential oil mixes, in addition to the use of individual oils, can be customized to produce one-of-a-kind atmosphere-enhancing experiences. Through the use of oils that have effects that are complementary to one another, it is possible to boost their total influence, which can result in more profound emotional benefits. Creating a rich, fragrant experience that strikes a balance between uplifting and anchoring properties can be accomplished, for instance, by combining citrus oils, ylang-ylang, and frankincense. In addition to enhancing mood, frankincense, which is well-known for its meditative qualities, can aid in relaxing the mind and make it easier to digest intense emotions. When it comes to fostering a sense of inner calm while simultaneously improving one's mental state, this combination is extremely useful for individuals.

Essential oils have a wide range of applications, which is one of the most fascinating elements of employing them to improve disposition. In order to make the atmosphere more uplifting, these oils can be included in a variety of facets of daily life. Taking a bath, for example, can be transformed into a calming ritual that promotes relaxation and increases mood by adding a few drops of citrus oil to the water before taking the bath. To a similar extent, the addition of essential oils to skincare regimes can confer an additional layer of psychological advantages. At the same time as it hydrates and nourishes the face, utilizing a facial mist that contains rose or geranium oil can be a great way to improve one's mood.

A growing number of people have become interested in the role that essential oils play in fostering emotional well-being in recent years as a result of the emergence of mindfulness and self-care practices. One way to improve the experience and strengthen one's connection to the here and now is to incorporate essential oils into mindfulness techniques like yoga or meditation. For the purpose of facilitating grounding and emotional clarity, meditation methods frequently make use of oils such as frankincense and sandalwood. Individuals are able to establish a more profound connection with their inner selves as a result of the calming scents that create an atmosphere that is conducive to relaxation and contemplation.

In addition, it is becoming increasingly clear that the psychological impacts of essential oils are supported by scientific studies. The beneficial effects of essential oils on one's mood and mental well-being have been established by a great number of previous research. By way of illustration, a study that included individuals who suffered from anxiety discovered that breathing lavender oil greatly decreased the amount of anxiety they experienced and improved their mood overall. The inhalation of bergamot oil was shown to result in a significant reduction in anxiety and an improvement in mood prior to the operation, according to a study that investigated the effects of aromatherapy on patients who were due to undergo surgery. These findings lend credence to the idea that essential oils have the ability to serve as indispensable instruments for increasing one's mood and emotional well-being.

Even if there are a lot of advantages to using essential oils to improve one's mood, it is vital to have a conscious and responsible approach to using them. Whenever choosing oils and blends, individuals ought to be conscious of their individual sensitivities and preferences. To verify that there are no adverse reactions, it is recommended to perform a patch test before using oils topically. In addition, in order to guarantee the efficacy and safety of essential oils, it is vital to select and purchase pure essential oils of the highest possible quality from trustworthy organizations.

Not only do essential oils have the ability to improve one's mood, but they can also help one heal emotionally by treating the underlying problems that are associated with negative moods. Individuals who are experiencing emotional turmoil as a result of hormonal fluctuations can benefit from the use of oils such as geranium and clary sage, which are known for their capacity to regulate mood swings and bring about a balance in hormones. Not only has it been demonstrated that geranium oil can alleviate symptoms of depression and anxiety, but it can also promote a sense of emotional stability and well-being.

In addition to fostering deeper connections with other people, the emotional benefits of essential oils can extend beyond the scope of the individual. The utilization of essential oils in social contexts has the potential to provide an environment that is more welcoming and upbeat, thereby increasing conversation and developing connections. The use of uplifting oils, for instance, in group situations, such as family get-togethers or social events, can help to foster sentiments of joy and unity among the attendees. Memories and connections that will last a lifetime can be formed via the shared experience of pleasant smells, which can assist in enabling open communication and emotional bonding.

It is becoming increasingly apparent that essential oils, which are natural treatments, offer a distinctive method of achieving emotional well-being as we continue to investigate the powerful benefits that essential oils have on mood enhancement. It is possible for individuals to cultivate a more positive emotional landscape and improve their overall quality of life by utilizing the power of scent and the therapeutic properties of oils together. It is a deeply personal journey that requires self-exploration and experimentation in order to find the oils and blends that make the best mood-enhancement products.

A life that is more balanced, joyful, and fulfilling can ultimately be achieved through the incorporation of essential oils into daily routines. Reminding oneself of the significance of self-care and emotional well-being can be accomplished through the rituals of inhaling, applying, and incorporating oils into a variety of practices. We are opening ourselves up to a world of possibilities when we acknowledge the potential of essential oils to improve our mood. We are letting the therapeutic gifts that nature has to offer direct us toward a more positive environment emotionally.

In conclusion, the utilization of essential oils for the purpose of enhancing one's mood is a method that successfully combines ancient knowledge and contemporary scientific understanding. A pathway is created for individuals who are looking to improve their overall well-being and lift their spirits by combining the therapeutic benefits of these oils with the powerful connection that exists between scent and emotions. Individuals can uncover the secrets of nature and build a stronger feeling of happiness, balance, and emotional resilience by studying the broad range of essential oils that are accessible and understanding the unique characteristics of each of these oils. It is without a doubt that the role of essential oils in fostering happy feelings and improving mood will continue to be vital as we continue to place a greater emphasis on mental health and well-being. Essential oils provide a method that is both natural and efficient for navigating the demands of contemporary life.

Sleep Improvement

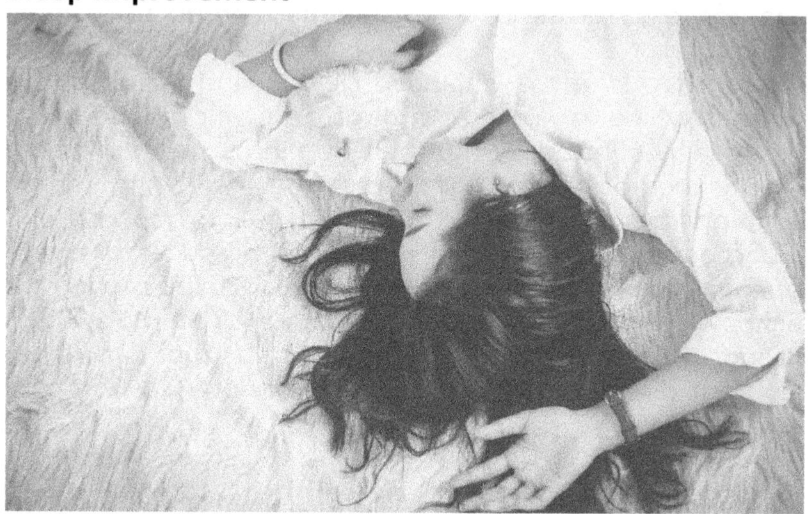

Enhancing one's quality of sleep is an essential component of total health and well-being, as it plays a significant part in three aspects of health: physical, mental, and emotional. In addition to having a substantial impact on our everyday functioning, mood, cognitive capacities, and even immune system performance, the quality and quantity of sleep we get have a huge impact. Natural therapies for improving sleep have garnered an increasing amount of attention in recent years, notably essential oils and oils derived from plants. As a result of their relaxing and sedative qualities, these natural chemicals have been consumed for ages across a variety of cultures. It is becoming increasingly clear that these oils can act as helpful instruments for improving the quality of sleep and encouraging relaxation as research continues to shed light on the advantages of these oils to a greater extent.

The human body has a complex relationship with sleep, which is managed by circadian rhythms, which are responsible for determining our shifts between sleep and wakefulness. We may have trouble going to sleep or remaining asleep if we interrupt these natural routines, which can be caused by stress, worry, or choices we make in our lifestyle. In addition to influencing the body's stress response, essential oils have been demonstrated to promote relaxation and generate an environment that is conducive to peaceful sleep. This is due to the specific chemical compositions of essential oils. Lavender oil is one of the oils that has been studied extensively for its potential to improve sleep quality. In addition to being well known for its calming floral aroma, lavender has been the subject of much research due to its sedative properties. Inhaling lavender oil has been shown to greatly increase the quality of sleep, minimize the number of things that disrupt sleep, and boost feelings of tranquility, according to research. Creating a state of relaxation that gets the body ready for sleep is mostly related to the oil's ability to drop blood pressure and heart rate, which in turn creates a state of relaxation.

A study that was conducted and published in the Journal of Medicinal Food found that participants who inhaled lavender oil before going to bed reported an improvement in the quality of their sleep as well as an increase in the total amount of time they spent sleeping. Additionally, it has been demonstrated that lavender oil can reduce levels of anxiety, making it an excellent option for individuals who struggle with mental racing or stress that prevents them from falling or staying asleep. In order to facilitate a more seamless transition into rest, the relaxing characteristics of lavender can assist folks in making the transition from the hectic activities of the day to a more relaxed state. Chamomile oil is yet another essential oil that has gained consideration due to the fact that it has the ability to improve sleep. Due to the relaxing properties that it has on the nervous system, chamomile has been utilized as a natural cure for a variety of disorders for several centuries. Compounds that support relaxation and enhance the quality of sleep are found in the oil that is extracted from chamomile flowers. An individual's ability to fall asleep more quickly and improve the overall quality of their sleep has been demonstrated by research. Those who have trouble falling asleep or staying asleep after a long and stressful day would benefit tremendously from this, for example.

A powerful sleep aid that has been used for generations to promote relaxation and increase sleep quality is oil extracted from the root of the valerian plant. As a result of its well-known capacity to alleviate anxiety and bring about a state of calm, Valerian is an ideal option for individuals who suffer racing thoughts whenever they are about to go to bed. The quality of sleep and the amount of time it takes to fall asleep have both been shown to be greatly improved by valerian oil, according to a number of studies. Valerian extract was found to be beneficial in reducing sleep latency and enhancing overall sleep quality in those who suffer from insomnia, according to a review that was published in the journal Sleep Medicine Reviews for the purpose of reporting its findings. Individuals are able to provide themselves with a calming atmosphere that encourages peaceful sleep and relaxation by introducing valerian oil into their evening routine.

There are a number of essential oils that have demonstrated the potential to improve the quality of sleep in addition to these well-known oils. Bergamot oil, which has a fragrance that is reminiscent of citrus fruits, has been discovered to alleviate feelings of anxiety and to encourage relaxation. Those who deal with sleep problems caused by anxiety may find that bergamot oil is a good alternative for them. According to a study that was published in the Journal of Clinical Psychology, bergamot oil has the ability to considerably reduce anxiety levels in those who suffer from stress-related diseases. The invigorating scent of bergamot has the ability to turn an environment into one that is soothing, which can assist in reducing the stress that is frequently associated with a busy mind.

Sandalwood oil is yet another essential oil that has the potential to provide support for the improvement of sleep. Since ancient times, people from many different cultures have relied on the calming effects of sandalwood, which is characterized by a scent that is both rich and woodsy. By influencing the body's production of serotonin, a neurotransmitter that plays a critical part in regulating sleep patterns, sandalwood oil has been proven to be effective in promoting relaxation and helping to improve the quality of sleep. Individuals are able to create a tranquil atmosphere that promotes healthy sleep throughout the night by introducing sandalwood oil into their evening routine.

It is possible to use essential oils in a variety of methods in order to improve one's sleep, which gives individuals the opportunity to identify the approach that is most effective for them. When it comes to using essential oils for sleep, inhalation is one of the most prevalent approaches. By incorporating a few drops of the selected oil into a diffuser, it is possible to achieve this goal so producing an atmosphere in the bedroom that is conducive to relaxation. In addition to filling the room with a nice perfume, diffusing essential oils enables the therapeutic chemicals to be inhaled, which not only helps to promote relaxation but also helps to get the mind ready for sleep. A personal inhaler can also be made by pouring a few drops of essential oil on a cotton ball and then inhaling the aroma before going to bed. This is another option for individuals who want it.

Using essential oils to increase the quality of sleep can also be accomplished through the medium of topical application. Essential oils are absorbed into the bloodstream when they are applied to the skin, which enables their ability to exert their medicinal effects.

Essential oils can be diluted in a carrier oil, such as sweet almond or jojoba oil, to make a sleep oil blend. This is a technique that is widely used. In order to induce relaxation and get the body ready for sleep, this mixture can be massaged onto pulse points, which include the wrists, the neck, and the temples. When combined, the calming aroma of essential oils with the soothing touch of massage can produce a powerful experience that contributes to improved sleep.

Another lovely technique to get the body ready for a good night's sleep is to take a shower or bath that is warm and infused with aromatic oils. It is possible to create a tranquil environment by adding a few drops of lavender, chamomile, or ylang-ylang oil to a warm bath. This will assist to relax the body as well as the mindset. After a hard day, it is much simpler to relax and unwind when you combine the benefits of warm water and calming aromas. This combination has the potential to greatly reduce stress and anxiety. It is possible to send a message to the body that it is time to wind down and get ready for sleep by using essential oils in a bedtime regimen that contains essential oils.

Additionally essential to enhancing the quality of one's sleep is the establishment of an atmosphere that is conducive to sleep. By utilizing aromatherapy candles, sprays, or reed diffusers, essential oils can be incorporated into the design of a particular bedroom. As a result of the peaceful ambiance that can be created by the aromas that fill the air, it is much simpler to relax and fall asleep while in this environment. Enhancing the whole experience can also be accomplished by combining the use of essential oils with other methods of relaxation, such as practicing meditation or deep breathing. It is possible to achieve a more profound sense of relaxation and a smoother transition into sleep by engaging in mindfulness practices while inhaling aromas that are calming.

In addition, it is vital to have an awareness of the power of regularity in order to improve the quality of bedtime sleep. People are able to develop good sleeping patterns by establishing a regular schedule for going to bed, which sends a message to the body that it is time to sleep. A reminder to put relaxation and self-care at the forefront of your routine can be provided by the incorporation of essential oils into this practice. Over time, the quality of sleep can be considerably improved by taking the time to relax, whether that be through the inhalation of relaxing scents, the practice of mild stretches, or participation in mindfulness exercises.

Additionally, it is vital to approach the use of essential oils with mindfulness and awareness despite the fact that they offer several benefits for the enhancement of sleep. When picking oils, individuals should be conscious of their individual sensitivities and preferences with regard to the oils they use. To verify that there are no adverse reactions, it is recommended to perform a patch test before using oils topically. In addition, in order to guarantee the efficacy and safety of essential oils, it is vital to select and purchase pure essential oils of the highest possible quality from trustworthy organizations. In addition, it is vital to utilize oils that have been diluted, particularly when applying them to the skin, in order to lessen the likelihood of irritation.

The mental well-being that essential oils can promote can indirectly lead to greater sleep, in addition to the sleep-enhancing characteristics that essential oils possess. As a result of their capacity to manage mood swings and maintain hormonal equilibrium, oils such as geranium and clary sage are beneficial for people who are experiencing emotional turmoil that may prevent them from falling or staying asleep. In particular, it has been demonstrated that geranium oil can produce a sense of emotional stability and decrease the symptoms of anxiety. An individual can develop a more holistic strategy for improving the quality of their sleep by addressing the emotional issues that contribute to sleep disruptions.

The increasing corpus of research that has been conducted on the usage of essential oils for the purpose of improving sleep quality provides evidence that these oils are effective as natural treatments. Several essential oils have been demonstrated to have a beneficial effect on sleep patterns, alleviate anxiety, and improve the overall quality of sleep, according to research reports. In a study that was published in the Journal of Clinical Sleep Medicine, for instance, the researchers discovered that individuals who used lavender oil had better quality sleep and fewer sleep disruptions than those who did not use the oil before bedtime. Essential oils have the potential to be useful tools for increasing sleep and fostering calm, as demonstrated by this research.

It is vital to note that the usefulness of essential oils with regard to improving sleep may vary from person to person when individuals investigate the benefits of essential oils for improving sleep. It is essential to explore and personalize one's approach because what is successful for one person might not necessarily be successful for another. This can help folks discover what resonates with them and lead to greater sleep quality. Keeping a sleep journal to track the effects of various oils and approaches might be helpful in this regard. People can get the ability to take care of their sleep health and develop individualized routines that are in line with their own requirements by going through this process of self-discovery.

The utilization of essential oils for the purpose of enhancing one's ability to sleep is, in conclusion, a harmonious combination of old knowledge and contemporary scientific research. In addition to their capacity to impact the body's stress response and to induce relaxation, the therapeutic effects of essential oils contribute to the creation of a pathway for persons who are looking for comfortable sleep. Individuals are able to build a more calm sleep environment, better their bedtime rituals, and eventually improve their entire well-being if they make use of the power of essential oils. The significance of essential oils in encouraging peaceful sleep will definitely continue to be crucial as we continue to place a greater emphasis on the importance of sleep health in a society that is becoming increasingly fast-paced. Essential oils provide a method that is both authentic and efficient for navigating the difficulties of modern living. The secrets to a better night's sleep, as well as the keys to reclaiming one's health and vigor, can be unlocked by individuals who embrace the power of nature's healing gifts.

CHAPTER V

Practical Applications in Everyday Life

Household Solutions

In recent years, there has been a resurgence of interest in natural treatments, such as essential oils and plant-based extracts, as alternatives to synthetic goods for various domestic uses. This interest has been especially prevalent in the United States. The increased awareness of health and environmental problems has been the driving force behind the transition away from chemical-based solutions and toward alternatives inspired by nature rather than chemicals. Essential oils are powerful compounds that can be utilized in a wide variety of ways within the home. They are obtained from various sections of plants, such as leaves, blossoms, seeds, and roots, and they offer both practicality and a link to the earth's old wisdom.

From a long time ago, it has been acknowledged that these oils possess therapeutic characteristics. On the other hand, a great number of individuals are just lately starting to find their versatility in day-to-day living, particularly as efficient remedies for domestic problems. Lavender, tea tree, eucalyptus, lemon, and rosemary oils are some examples of oils that can be used to substitute harsh chemicals for cleaning, personal care, pest control, and air purification. These oils have benefits that are just as potent, if not more so, than those of the chemicals. Understanding how to make use of their natural qualities for a variety of applications is one of the most important things to do.

Cleaning is one of the most common applications for oils, one of the most common uses of oils. When used for an extended period of time, household cleaning products frequently include a combination of chemicals that have the potential to irritate the skin, create respiratory problems, or trigger allergic reactions. Essential oils, on the other hand, offer a natural and environmentally respectful option. Because of their powerful antimicrobial and antibacterial qualities, oils like lemon, tea tree, and eucalyptus are an excellent choice for sanitizing surfaces, worktops, and floors. Not only do these oils clean effectively, but they also leave behind an aroma that is completely natural and fresh. As an example, a straightforward mixture consisting of water, vinegar, and a few drops of lemon oil can be utilized as an all-purpose cleaner. This mixture is capable of removing grease and filth while also acting as an odor-neutralizer.

Particularly praised for its antifungal and antibacterial characteristics is tea tree oil, which has been recommended for use. Mold is a big problem that can be a substantial concern in wet areas of the house, such as bathrooms and basements. It is a powerful ally in the fight against mold. It is possible to prevent the growth of mold by spraying a solution consisting of water, vinegar, and tea tree oil directly on surfaces that are contaminated with mold. This is an alternative to chemical mold removers that are both natural and effective. In a similar manner, eucalyptus oil can be utilized to clean surfaces while also imparting an aroma that is both revitalizing and energizing.

Essential oils are increasingly being used for a variety of purposes, including cleaning and air purification. The release of volatile organic compounds (VOCs) into the air by a large number of commercial air fresheners and candles is a factor that can contribute to the pollution of the air inside buildings and may be detrimental to respiratory health. Aromatherapy with essential oils, such as lavender, peppermint, or citrus oils, can naturally clean and purify the air, thereby lowering the number of bacteria and viruses that are carried through the air while also creating an ambiance that is pleasant and peaceful. If you want to refresh a space without the potentially dangerous side effects of synthetic perfumes, you can use a few drops of oil in a diffuser or add it to water in a spray bottle on your window.

In the realm of pest control, essential oils are also becoming increasingly popular. The potent aromas of some oils are effective at warding off a wide variety of pests, including spiders, ants, and mosquitoes of various kinds. For instance, while citronella oil has been used for a very long time to ward off mosquitoes, peppermint oil is a natural repellent that can be used against mice and other insects. It is easy to make homemade repellents by utilizing essential oils, and they can be just as powerful as ones purchased from the shop. However, they do not contain any additional chemicals that could be harmful to animals or children under the age of five. When applied to places that are prone to pests, a mixture of water, witch hazel, and essential oils can be sprayed to provide natural and risk-free protection against unwanted intruders.

Personal care is another area in which essential oils offer a wide variety of answers when it comes to household problems. Essential oils can be used to make handmade lotions, shampoos, and soaps that are kind to the skin and good for the environment. This is an alternative to using products that are loaded with chemicals. As a result of the calming and soothing effects that oils like lavender and chamomile are known to possess, these oils are wonderful complements to skin lotions, massage oils, and bath salts. Essential oils, when incorporated into DIY skincare routines, have the potential to alleviate irritation and promote healing without exposing the skin to synthetic chemicals. This is especially beneficial for individuals experiencing sensitive skin.

Using essential oils to make hand sanitizers at home is a common home remedy that is very popular. The usage of hand sanitizers has become increasingly common in contemporary homes, particularly in light of the increased emphasis placed on hygiene in recent years. Regrettably, many of the versions that are sold in stores contain alcohol and other drying ingredients, which can cause the skin to lose its natural oils. An excellent hand sanitizer that kills bacteria without leaving hands feeling dry or irritated can be made by combining tea tree oil or lavender oil with aloe vera gel. This combination ensures that the hand sanitizer is both hydrating and effective.

Laundry care is another area in which essential oils can be of great assistance. Laundry detergents and fabric softeners used in commercial establishments frequently contain perfumes and chemicals that have the potential to stay on garments and cause skin irritation. Lavender, lemon, and eucalyptus essential oils are some examples of essential oils that can be used in homemade laundry detergents or used in dryer balls to impart a natural fragrance to linens and garments. The antibacterial and antimicrobial qualities of these oils, in addition to the fact that they impart a pleasant aroma, contribute to the enhanced cleaning capabilities of laundry regimens.

Essential oils can be utilized in the kitchen for a variety of purposes, including cooking and the preservation of food. When used in moderation, oils such as lemon, basil, rosemary, and oregano have the ability to impart a sense of depth and taste to foods. For culinary reasons, however, it is absolutely necessary to make use of essential oils that are of food-grade quality, as certain oils are not suitable for consumption. Because these concentrated oils have the potential to impart a fragrance that is more powerful than that of dried herbs and spices, they are an invaluable asset to any kitchen. Furthermore, due to the antibacterial capabilities that they possess, distinct essential oils have the potential to be utilized as natural preservatives. As an illustration, thyme and clove oil have the ability to limit the growth of bacteria, which in turn helps to extend the shelf life of foods.

Additionally, essential oils have a role in the garden, where they can improve the health of plants and provide a natural means of controlling diseases. Without the use of chemical pesticides, plants can be protected from aphids, mites, and other pests by spraying them with a solution of water and neem oil. This solution can be used to spray on plants. Additionally, scents such as lavender and rosemary have the ability to attract helpful insects such as bees and butterflies, which in turn promotes pollination and overall garden health. Essential oils provide a sustainable and chemical-free alternative for gardeners who are concerned about the environment and want to keep their plants flourishing.

The advantages of essential oils extend even farther into the realm of mental and emotional well-being, which can have an effect on the ambiance of the home. Research has demonstrated that aromatherapy, which involves the utilization of essential oils for the purpose of emotional and psychological healing, can effectively alleviate stress, enhance mood, and facilitate relaxation. When applied to pillows, a few drops of lavender oil can help to promote a pleasant night's sleep. On the other hand, diffusing citrus oils can help to revitalize and boost the spirit during the day. Aromatherapy is a good method for achieving a balance between the practical parts of household maintenance and the fostering of mental wellness. This can be accomplished by helping to create a quiet environment within the home.

Essential oils, in addition to their direct use, are in line with a broader commitment to sustainability and environmental responsibility. The transition away from synthetic goods and toward oils derived from plants is a manifestation of a growing desire to limit the impact that household consumption has on the environment and to reduce levels of chemical exposure. Essential oils are a sustainable option for consumers who are concerned about the environment because many of them are sourced from plant sources that can be replenished. In addition, homes can make a contribution to the reduction of trash and the promotion of a more sustainable way of life by decreasing their reliance on plastic bottles and packaging from commercial products that are designed for single use.

On the other hand, it is absolutely necessary to approach the utilization of essential oils with caution and reverence. The potency of essential oils necessitates that they be diluted prior to their application in order to prevent skin irritation or other undesirable effects. In addition, there are some oils that are not suitable for use by small children or animals. Therefore, it is essential to conduct research and adhere to the rules for safe application. Essential oils have a long shelf life when they are handled correctly, which makes them an economical alternative for a variety of requirements that are found in the home.

It is actually astonishing how versatile essential oils are when it comes to their use as home solutions. In addition to providing natural and efficient alternatives to items that are loaded with chemicals, they contribute to a healthier environment and home. Essential oils offer a wide range of applications that can improve an individual's day-to-day life, including but not limited to cleaning, personal care, air purification, and pest control. Individuals are reconnected with the curative capabilities of plants that have been utilized for millennia as a result of their incorporation into contemporary households, which represents a return to the wisdom of nature.

Individuals not only enhance their own personal health but also contribute to a lifestyle that is more sustainable and environmentally friendly when they incorporate essential oils into their regular routines at home. The natural power of these oils has the potential to convert the home into a sanctuary of well-being, cleanliness, and calmness, where the connection between nature and everyday living is cherished and respected. We have the ability to unlock the mysteries of nature and harness its power for the purpose of creating a better and healthier world via the attentive and informed use of essential oils.

Personal Care and Wellness

Essential oils provide a safe and efficient substitute for synthetic products, which is why they are becoming more and more important in health and personal care regimens. These powerful chemical components are contained in these plant-derived oils, which have been utilized for ages in cosmetic and medicinal procedures. When it comes to promoting physical, mental, and even spiritual well-being, essential oils stand out in today's world when there is a rising desire for natural and holistic methods of self-care. Because of their adaptability, they can be used in a variety of personal care applications, such as skin care, mental health, and even spiritual activities.

Essential oils are a significant component of skincare products because of their numerous therapeutic benefits. The largest organ in the body, the skin, is continually subjected to harmful UV radiation, environmental pollutants, and the aging process itself, all of which can cause damage and hasten the aging process. Although a lot of commercial skincare products aim to address these problems, they frequently contain ingredients that, in the long run, may cause more harm than benefit. Conversely, essential oils offer a safe, all-natural remedy that promotes skin health without having any negative side effects. Essential oils like rosehip, tea tree, and lavender have become commonplace in many people's skincare routines.

Due to its well-known ability to calm and soothe, lavender oil is perfect for sensitive or irritated skin. It's a fantastic option for treating acne and other skin irritations because of its anti-inflammatory and antibacterial properties. Using lavender oil on a regular basis can help relieve burns, lessen redness, and even stop scarring. Its calming properties also aid in emotional well-being by reducing stress and anxiety, both of which can negatively affect the condition of the skin. Including lavender in a regular skincare regimen is beneficial for the skin as well as for general relaxation and well-being.

Another well-liked essential oil for skin care is tea tree oil, especially for oily and acne-prone skin. Its potent antibacterial and antifungal qualities aid in combating the germs responsible for acne, and its capacity to regulate sebum production makes it a preferred choice for individuals experiencing breakouts. Tea tree oil softly cleanses the face without irritating or drying it out, in contrast to aggressive acne treatments that can strip the skin of its natural oils. Tea tree oil is very strong. Therefore, it's best to dilute it with a carrier oil before putting it directly on the skin to avoid irritation.

Even though rosehip oil is essentially a carrier oil, its advantages are frequently increased by adding essential oils to it. It has a lot of antioxidants and important fatty acids, which promote skin suppleness, scar reduction, and skin cell regeneration. Rosehip oil may make a potent combination with anti-aging essential oils like geranium or frankincense that nourishes the skin, minimizes the look of fine wrinkles, and encourages a young complexion. These kinds of oil blends combine the restorative qualities of carrier oils with the medicinal advantages of essential oils to provide a comprehensive approach to skincare.

Essential oils are becoming a common option for hair care in addition to skincare. Numerous stresses, including heat styling, chemical treatments, and environmental conditions, can cause damage to hair and even cause hair loss. Synthetic compounds found in many hair care treatments can deplete hair of its natural oils, leaving it brittle and dry. Essential oils offer a natural means of strengthening the hair shaft, nourishing the scalp, and enhancing general hair health.

The capacity of rosemary oil to promote hair development and enhance scalp circulation is widely recognized. By rubbing rosemary oil into the scalp, either undiluted or blended with another oil, people can lessen dry scalp and dandruff and encourage healthier, fuller hair. It is also useful in preventing premature graying and hair loss due to its stimulating qualities. Another great option for hair care is peppermint oil, which has cooling and stimulating properties that assist in increasing blood flow to the scalp and encourage the growth of healthy hair. It also helps to balance oil production and soothes dry, itchy scalps.

Additionally, essential oils can be utilized to make conditioners, serums, and scalp treatments—all-natural substitutes for salon-quality hair treatments. For example, a nourishing hair mask that adds moisture and luster to dry, damaged hair can be made with a mixture of lavender oil and argan oil. Additionally, to encourage hair development and lessen hair loss brought on by stress or hormone imbalances, oils like cedarwood and clary sage can be added to scalp treatments.

Essential oils are highly valued in the field of body care because of their capacity to both nourish and revitalize the skin and offer therapeutic advantages. Sweet almond, coconut, and jojoba oils are frequently used as carrier oils in body moisturizers because they offer intense moisture without blocking pores. These mixes can provide extra advantages, including relieving tense muscles, lowering inflammation, and encouraging relaxation when paired with essential oils.

To ease joint and muscular pain, eucalyptus oil, which has anti-inflammatory and pain-relieving qualities, can be mixed with body lotion or massage oil. A cooling combination of peppermint and eucalyptus oil helps relieve tight muscles and hasten recuperation after exercise. In contrast, chamomile oil is well-known for its relaxing properties and is frequently utilized in body care products to lessen inflammation, redness, and irritation of the skin. Its mild composition makes it perfect for delicate skin types, and its pleasant, herbal aroma encourages unwinding and alleviating tension.

An additional method to include natural goods in a personal care regimen is through the use of deodorants formulated with essential oils. Aluminum and other synthetic components found in many traditional deodorants have the potential to be detrimental to the body, particularly when applied close to lymph nodes. Essential oils with inherent antibacterial qualities, such as tea tree, lavender, and lemongrass, are useful in dispelling microorganisms that cause odors. Essential oils can be used with natural materials like coconut oil and baking soda to make an excellent deodorant that is free of chemicals and nourishes the skin while preventing odors.

Another location where essential oils excel is in the bath, where they offer a posh and healing experience. An average bath can be transformed into a calming, spa-like experience by adding a few drops of essential oils to the water. Oils that encourage relaxation and sound sleep, such as lavender, chamomile, and sandalwood, are ideal for making a soothing bath. Conversely, stimulating oils such as rosemary, eucalyptus, and peppermint can be used to make an invigorating and refreshing bath that awakens the senses and helps to declutter the mind.

These oils are beneficial to the body, but they also produce a rich, aromatic atmosphere that improves well-being all around.

One of the most popular uses for essential oils is aromatherapy, which is important for wellness and self-care. Essential oils can directly affect mood, emotions, and cognitive function by inhalation. Essential oils can be applied topically, added to a bath, or diffused to assist in reducing tension, anxiety, and sadness. The limbic system, which controls emotions and memory, is stimulated by the aroma of essential oils, which is how aromatherapy works scientifically.

For example, lavender oil is well renowned for its ability to calm and relax people. It is frequently used in aromatherapy to ease anxiety, encourage calm sleep, and lower stress levels. Before going to bed, inhaling lavender oil can assist in promoting pleasant surroundings and better quality sleep. Similar to this, oils with mood-enhancing qualities include bergamot, clary sage, and ylang-ylang. These oils can help reduce emotions of despair, anxiety, and emotional imbalance.

On the other hand, oils that promote mental clarity, attention, and alertness include peppermint and rosemary. Particularly peppermint oil is well-known for its energizing aroma, which aids in reducing mental weariness and enhancing focus. It is frequently used in aromatherapy to increase vitality and enhance mental clarity. Another potent essential oil that has been demonstrated to improve memory and cognitive function is rosemary oil, which is why people who need to concentrate on difficult activities or are students often use it.

Essential oils are employed in spiritual and mindfulness practices in addition to their medical and emotional advantages. Many people use essential oils in their prayer, yoga, and meditation practices in order to improve focus, provide a sense of grounding, and strengthen their spiritual ties. Because of their centering and grounding qualities, oils like patchouli, sandalwood, and frankincense are frequently employed. These oils are said to heighten meditation, foster spiritual awareness, and foster inner balance and tranquility. These oils can be used to elevate meditation by diffusing them throughout the practice or applying them to certain pulse spots.

Chakra balancing and other energy healing techniques like Reiki also use essential oils. Every essential oil is thought to be associated with a certain chakra, or energy point, within the body. For example, the crown chakra, which is in charge of enlightenment and spiritual connection, is frequently linked to frankincense and sandalwood. When used in chakra-balancing exercises, these oils can aid in opening and aligning the crown chakra, which fosters purpose and spiritual awareness. Similarly, the third eye chakra, which is in charge of inner understanding and intuition, is linked to oils like lavender and clary sage.

Another option to include essential oils in a personal care routine is to create customized oil mixes for particular emotional or physical requirements. People can develop personalized treatments for a variety of issues, including pain management, skin care, and stress and relaxation, by combining different oils according to their medicinal qualities. For instance, a combination of chamomile, bergamot, and lavender can produce a serene ambiance that's ideal for winding down after a demanding day. However, a combination of eucalyptus, lemon, and peppermint can create an atmosphere that is stimulating and upbeat, which is perfect for increasing focus and energy.

Essential oils are frequently utilized in massage therapy to increase the therapeutic effects of the procedure. Essential oil-infused massage oils can ease soreness, lessen inflammation, and encourage relaxation. Because of their relaxing and pain-relieving qualities, oils, including chamomile, lavender, and marjoram, are frequently used in massage therapy. The body and mind benefit from the calming massage that these essential oils provide when mixed with a carrier oil such as jojoba or sweet almond. When massage treatment is paired with essential oils' therapeutic qualities, it provides a comprehensive approach to well-being that promotes both mental and physical health.

Lastly, personal care items like scrubs, lotions, and perfumes can also be made with essential oils. People can create signature perfumes that are a reflection of their likes and personalities by blending different essential oils. In addition to having a lovely scent, these natural perfumes offer the medicinal properties of the oils they contain. For instance, a perfume including sandalwood, ylang-ylang, and jasmine can produce a seductive, calming scent that encourages emotional balance and relaxation. In a similar vein, a lotion enriched with rose, chamomile, and lavender oil can soothe the skin and senses while offering intense moisture.

In summary, essential oils can be used for a variety of personal care and wellness tasks, such as emotional balance, spiritual activities, and hair and skincare maintenance. Their natural and therapeutic qualities, along with their versatility, make them a priceless tool for anybody looking for a comprehensive approach to self-care. People can enjoy the lovely and aromatic effects of these potent plant extracts as well as improve their physical, emotional, and spiritual well-being by introducing essential oils into their everyday routines. Essential oils are becoming more and more popular, and with it, so will their significance in personal care and well-being. They provide a safe and practical option for anyone looking to lead a more balanced, healthy lifestyle.

Creating Personalized Oil Blends

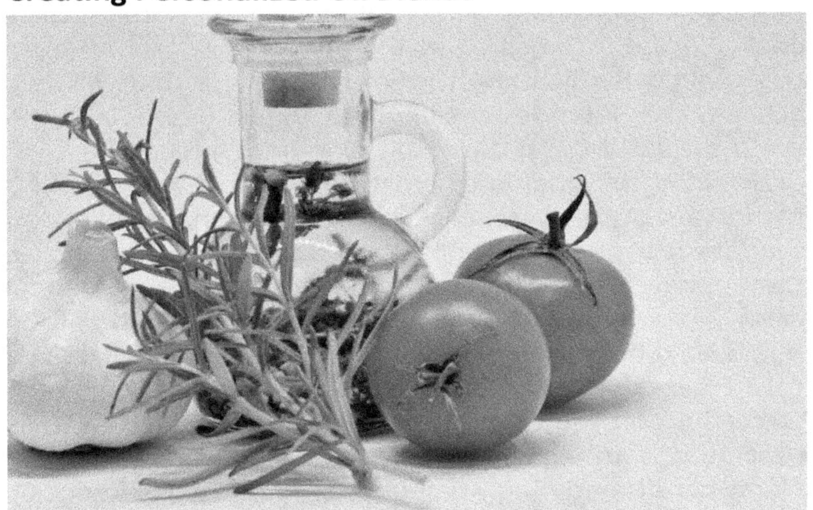

People can fully explore the potential of essential oils by making customized oil blends that cater to their unique emotional, physical, and spiritual needs. The dynamic process of blending essential oils involves giving careful thought to each oil's distinct qualities, aroma, and therapeutic effects. This is both an art and a science. This method transcends basic aromatherapy and becomes an immersive experience in which each blend represents the person's preferences, goals, and personality.

It's crucial to start with a knowledge of essential oils in order to comprehend how to make customized oil blends. Essential oils are extremely potent plant extracts, and each one has a distinct set of chemical characteristics that provide particular advantages. These advantages might include everything from mental health, like lowering stress levels or encouraging relaxation, to physical healing, like releasing headaches or easing tense muscles. Because of this, when making an oil blend, you have to choose oils whose qualities complement the mix's intended use.

The first step in the procedure is to determine the blend's purpose. People usually mix oils for various goals; these could include skincare, invigorating, relaxing, or even therapeutic. By directing the selection of oils that will help achieve the intended result, this initial phase lays the groundwork for the entire blending procedure. For example, if the goal is to create a calming and soothing blend to reduce stress, oils like lavender, chamomile, and sandalwood might be ideal choices. Alternatively, for a more energizing blend to enhance focus and mental clarity, oils such as peppermint, rosemary, and lemon might be more appropriate.

Once the purpose of the blend has been determined, the next step is to explore the fragrance profiles of the oils being considered. Each essential oil belongs to a specific aromatic family, and the way these oils interact when blended together will significantly impact the overall scent. Understanding the different categories of oils, such as citrus, floral, woody, or spicy, helps ensure that the final blend is harmonious and pleasant to the senses. Citrus oils, for example, like lemon and orange, are often refreshing and uplifting, while floral oils like rose or jasmine can provide a soothing and calming effect. Woody oils such as cedarwood and sandalwood are frequently grounding and regulating, while spicy oils like cinnamon or clove can offer warmth and depth to a blend.

The process of blending oils entails understanding the concept of top, middle, and base notes, which is adapted from the perfume business. Each oil is classed as a top, middle, or base note, depending on how rapidly its aroma fades. Top notes, such as citrus oils like lemon or bergamot, are the most volatile, delivering the initial burst of scent but disappearing fast. Middle notes, such as lavender or rosemary, comprise the center of the combination and bring balance and depth. Base notes, like as patchouli or sandalwood, are the longest-lasting and offer depth and structure to the blend. A well-balanced combination often comprises oils from all three groups, giving a layered aroma that changes with time.

The amounts of oils in a blend are another significant issue. While there are no precise guidelines, a common ratio for blending essential oils is 30% top notes, 50% middle notes, and 20% base notes. These percentages can be changed, though, based on the blend's intended application and personal preferences. To achieve a calming blend for the evening, one could, for instance, add more base notes, such as frankincense or sandalwood, which have sedative qualities and aid in encouraging sound sleep.

The oils are mixed in small amounts to test the aroma after the oils have been chosen and the ratios have been established. Before making any last modifications, it's crucial to let the mix lie for at least 24 hours because essential oils can change in aroma as they interact and evaporate. This time of waiting enables the oils to integrate and reveal the blend's actual character. To balance the blend, add more of one oil or another as needed to make modifications.

Essential oils are frequently diluted with carrier oils to make them suitable for topical application. Because essential oils are so concentrated, applying them straight on the skin may irritate it. It is common practice to dilute essential oils while preserving their medicinal qualities by using carrier oils, such as jojoba, almond, or coconut oil. Because each carrier oil has a unique combination of advantageous qualities, the choice of carrier oil can also affect the blend's overall effectiveness. For instance, coconut oil has antibacterial qualities and is perfect for blends meant to soothe inflamed skin, while jojoba oil is well-known for its hydrating benefits and is frequently included in skincare products.

The creation of customized oil mixes is frequently motivated by the desire to promote emotional health.

Essential oils are a safe and natural approach to treat stress, anxiety, and depression. It is widely known that aroma has the ability to influence mood and emotions. Oils with relaxing and sedative properties, like bergamot, lavender, and chamomile, are frequently used in blends intended to encourage relaxation. On the other hand, combinations that are known to promote mental clarity and focus, such as peppermint, lemon, and rosemary, may be considered energetic.

Understanding how essential oils affect the limbic system—the area of the brain in charge of regulating emotions—is necessary when blending them for emotional support, as opposed to just making a pleasant scent. Essential oils stimulate the limbic system when inhaled, which aids with mood, memory, and behavior regulation. For instance, studies have demonstrated that lavender oil lowers cortisol levels, which helps reduce stress and anxiety, and that rosemary oil enhances memory retention and cognitive function.

Personalized oil mixes can be used not just for emotional support but also for physical illnesses. Many essential oils are perfect for crafting mixes that promote physical healing since they include anti-inflammatory, analgesic, and antibacterial qualities. For instance, clearing lung congestion and encouraging clear breathing can be achieved with a combination of eucalyptus, peppermint, and lavender. In a similar vein, a mixture of fennel, ginger, and peppermint might help with digestive problems, including bloating or nausea. It's crucial to take into account each oil's unique therapeutic qualities as well as how they complement one another to address the problem at hand when blending oils for physical health.

Another area where customized oil blends can have a big influence is skincare. Using essential oils, many people make their own skincare products as a natural substitute for store-bought beauty products. From fine lines and wrinkles to eczema and acne, essential oils can be utilized to treat a wide range of skin issues. For instance, tea tree oil, which has antibacterial qualities, is frequently included in mixtures intended to treat skin prone to acne. Tea tree oil can be used to make a potent acne-fighting mixture with oils that have anti-inflammatory and skin-regenerating qualities, such as lavender and frankincense.

Oils that assist encourage cell regeneration and increase skin suppleness, such as carrot seed, rosehip, and frankincense, are frequently included in anti-aging mixes. These oils can be mixed with hydrating carrier oils, such as jojoba or argan oil, to make a nourishing and revitalizing serum that encourages skin that is vibrant and youthful. Gentle oils, such as calendula or chamomile, can be added to the mixture to help relieve irritation and reduce inflammation in people with sensitive skin.

Blends of essential oils can benefit spiritual and mindfulness activities in addition to cosmetics and physical wellness. Since the fragrant properties of essential oils aid in establishing a sense of centering and focus, many people use them to enhance their yoga, meditation, or prayer. Because of their ability to center and ground, oils such as frankincense, patchouli, and sandalwood are frequently used to foster inner serenity and spiritual awareness. To create a spiritual and peaceful atmosphere, these oils can be applied to pulse points or diffused in a meditation place.

Essential oils are commonly utilized in energy healing modalities such as Reiki and chakra balancing in order to facilitate the healing process. It is thought that each essential oil has a corresponding chakra, or energy center, in the body and that these centers can be balanced and aligned by application. For instance, the crown chakra, which controls spiritual connection, is frequently related to frankincense and sandalwood, but the third eye chakra, which controls intuition and inner wisdom, is linked to lavender and clary sage.

Individuals can customize their spiritual practices by making customized oil mixes according to their aspirations and objectives. For example, frankincense, sandalwood, and myrrh, which are recognized for their grounding and spiritual qualities, could be included in a blend created to improve meditation. As an alternative, a mix with the heart-opening and emotionally balancing properties of rose, ylang-ylang, and geranium might be used to support emotional recovery.

Essential oils provide countless opportunities for crafting personalized mixtures that address the specific requirements of those who prefer producing their own personal care products. Essential oils can be used to make a wide range of natural and efficient personal care products, from body lotions and perfumes to hair treatments and bath oils. For instance, a unique perfume blend can have a foundation of sandalwood or vanilla with flower oils like jasmine and rose for further depth. Comparably, calming essential oils like chamomile and lavender might be blended with hydrating carrier oils like coconut or jojoba oil to create a body lotion.

Making customized oil blends is a creative and rewarding process in addition to being a useful skill. By experimenting with various combinations to find what works best for them, people can connect with their own intuition and creativity via the act of blending oils. Making customized blends is a very fulfilling and intimate procedure because each blend is a special representation of the person's requirements, preferences, and aspirations.

To sum up, the skill of crafting customized oil mixes enables people to fully utilize essential oils by customizing their application to fit particular emotional, physical, and spiritual requirements. Essential oils are a safe, natural approach to improving well-being and encourage harmony and balance in daily life, whether they are used for skin care, emotional support, physical healing, or spiritual practices. The options for generating custom blends are virtually endless as people become more aware of the medicinal benefits of essential oils and the distinctive ways in which they may be combined. Anyone can set out on a path of self-discovery and healing by experimenting, trusting their intuition, and learning a great deal about the oils themselves. By utilizing nature's power, they can craft custom blends that speak to their own distinct personalities.

CONCLUSION

As we come to the end of the book "Unlocking Nature's Secrets: The Power of Oils: Ancient Remedies for Modern Living," it becomes abundantly clear that essential oils are not merely a passing fad; rather, they are a significant part of the modern world. They are a bridge that connects us to the health-giving power of nature, representing the convergence of ancient knowledge and contemporary scientific understanding. Essential oils continue to play an important part in supporting our physical, emotional, and spiritual well-being, from their historical roots in ancient civilizations to their expanding presence in today's wellness practices. This is because essential oils have been used for centuries.

In this book, not only has the origins and use of essential oils in ancient cultures been investigated, but also the scientific rationale underlying the effectiveness of these oils has been discussed. On a molecular level, the natural components that are included inside essential oils interact with our bodies, providing a variety of advantages that range from the alleviation of pain to the enhancement of mood, from improved skin health to greater mental clarity. The utilization of essential oils is becoming increasingly incorporated into more integrative approaches to health and wellness as scientific research continues to corroborate what ancient cultures have known for thousands of years.

The fact that essential oils provide a comprehensive approach to health is one of the most important things that I have learned from this trip. In contrast to the majority of contemporary treatments, which focus on a single symptom or illness, oils are effective on numerous levels, healing the mind, body, and spirit. They offer a natural approach to improving well-being that does not involve the harsh side effects that are associated with synthetic drugs. Essential oils provide a wide range of solutions that are easy to get and versatile, making them an excellent choice for anyone looking for a way to alleviate stress, strengthen their immune system, or make their environment more calm.

Throughout the course of this book, we have had the opportunity to observe how oils can be utilized in a variety of elements of daily life, ranging from personal care and beauty routines to aromatherapy and cleaning the house. We are able to adopt a lifestyle that is more balanced, thoughtful, and health-conscious if we include these ancient treatments in our modern way of life. All individuals who are interested in enhancing their well-being in a natural way will find essential oils to be an appealing option because of their accessibility. The availability of a wide range of oil variations and the ease with which they may be applied make it possible to find an oil that meets any requirement.

It is important to note that with tremendous power comes the responsibility of using essential oils in a responsible and secure manner. It has been emphasized throughout this book how important it is to have a solid understanding of how to correctly dilute and apply oils, particularly when oil is being used for therapeutic purposes. It is necessary to have a thorough understanding of the specific features of each oil in order to prevent any unfavorable responses and to guarantee that you are making the most of the oils' capabilities. One of the stepping stones that will allow you to explore essential oils in a manner that is tailored to your specific requirements is the guidance on safe usage and customization that is included in this book.

When we consider the future, we see that the potential of essential oils is and will continue to be enormous and promising. It is expected that oils will continue to play a part in the pursuit of natural and holistic health as the wellness industry continues to engage in more research and innovation. Because of their adaptability and the fact that they have a long and illustrious history, essential oils will continue to be an invaluable resource for people who are looking to achieve harmony in both their physical and mental states.

Ultimately, "Unlocking Nature's Secrets" is not only a guide to essential oils; rather, it is an invitation to reestablish a harmonious relationship with the natural world. This is the conclusion of the book. We are able to have access to a source of healing and well-being that has been around for generations when we embrace the power of oils. This source has the potential to keep us well and happy. Please allow this information to motivate you to live in peace with the natural world and to make meaningful use of the treasures that it bestows upon you in order to enrich your life.

Thank you for buying and reading/ listening to our book. If you found this book useful/ helpful please take a few minutes and leave a review on the platform where you purchased our book. Your feedback matters greatly to us.